Stop Putting Yourself Last: The Self-Care Book For Moms

Be the Best Mom AND Live the Life You Want

Zoe Madden

ISBN 978-0-6452376-2-7

CONTENTS

Introduction   vii

1. SELF-CARE MAKES YOU AN (EVEN MORE)   1
AWESOME MOM
Take Care of Yourself   4
Chapter Takeaways   5

2. SLEEP YOUR WAY TO BEING THE BEST MOM   7
Why Is Sleep So Important?   8
How Do I Get a Good Night's Sleep?   9
Create the Optimum Sleep Environment   10
Watch What You Eat and Drink   12
Weighted Blankets   14
Sleep Cycles   14
Sleep Apnea   15
Chapter Takeaways   17

3. LOOK AFTER YOUR MIND (AND MAKE SURE IT   19
LOOKS AFTER YOU)
Overthinking   20
What Causes Overthinking?   21
How to Stop Overthinking   22
Living in the Present   24
Chapter Takeaways   24

4. KILL THE STRESS BEFORE IT KILLS YOU   27
Relieving Stress   28
Supplements for Stress Relief   35
Foods to Avoid When You're Stressed   40
Digital Detox, Self-Love And Reaching Out   41
Chapter Takeaways   43

5. BREATHE YOUR WAY TO SANITY   45
Still Your Mind   45
Calm Your Nervous System   47
Mindfulness   48
Meditation   51
Movement   54

Yoga   55
Chapter Takeaways   56

6. EAT FOR YOUR LIFE   57
So What is Healthy Eating?   58
Foods to Avoid   59
Planning Meals   63
Gluten   64
Keep Red Meat to a Minimum   66
Be Wary of Dairy   67
Avoid Unwanted Chemicals   67
Eat More Raw Fruits and Vegetables   70
Eating Organic   71
Hints From the Mediterranean Diet   72
Pinpoint Foods Your Body Doesn't Like   73
Your Health is in Your Hands   73
Chapter Takeaways   74

7. MOVE THAT BODY MAMA   75
Set Goals   76
Measure Progress   77
Use Social Media   77
How to Include Exercise in Your Busy Schedule   79
Chapter Takeaways   80

8. ALWAYS REMEMBER: YOU ARE IMPERFECTLY PERFECT   83
Love Your Body   83
Three Rules to Live By   84
Tips to Cultivate a Positive Attitude   87
Chapter Takeaways   88

9. SOCIAL CONNECTION IS A BASIC HUMAN NEED   91
Ways To Connect   92
Meeting New People   93
Connect with Your Partner   94
Chapter Takeaways   95

10. SIMPLIFY AND SMELL THE ROSES   97
Chapter Takeaways   99

Afterword   101
References   103
About the Author   107
Coming Soon   109

INTRODUCTION

Being a mom is hard! You get no sleep or time for yourself, and don't forget about the changes that you experience when you become a mom. I'm not talking about the physical changes—though it would be nice to get rid of those stretch marks—but the mental and emotional changes that come with it.

When you become a mom, you get advice from everyone, even the old lady standing behind you in the checkout line. But they never tell you how isolating it is. They don't tell you how often you'll lose your cool and how close to the edge you'll stand before you're ready to snap.

Now, add in the other moms you see on Facebook or television who look like they have themselves together. The camera doesn't lie? I call bull on that one. Just how hard did that mother scrub her house before taking that picture and posting it online? Don't even get me started on television moms—they're faker than Kim Kardashian's butt! The worst part is that this leaves regular moms feeling like a failure as a parent.

As a mother, you are often expected to do everything in the house, make sure everyone is safe, that their basic needs are met, and even manage everyone's emotions for them. Keep this up for long enough, and you can end up feeling burned out. Your lack of energy is not just a result of how hard you work, but is also a consequence of you trying to reach the unreachable expectations of mothers. Added to this, it can feel as if you're not expected to sleep or care about yourself at all. And you're always on call.

If you wake up every morning in a daze and operate on autopilot with no thought about who you are, what you need, and how your life is, you may well be on the path to burnout—which is why you need this book.

Before we continue, let's get one thing straight: self-care is not being selfish or self-indulgent. Self-care is simply looking after yourself mentally, physically, emotionally and spiritually so you can do everything you need to do in your life.

Self-care is about reawakening that part of yourself which has become lost, ignored, and forgotten from the beginning of motherhood. When was the last time you thought about truly living or paid any attention to your emotions? When did you last take some time just to enjoy yourself without feeling guilty or letting responsibility weigh you down?

Left unchecked, not looking after yourself will leave you feeling like a shell of the person you once were. We give up so much of ourselves when we become mothers that we have nothing left at the end of it all. You don't want to be the person who wakes up one day and realizes you have spent your entire life letting it go by.

We expect mothers to live for their children, but that's just a dangerous myth. You are a person in your own right, and you also need recognition and love.

It's important you deal with the stress. If you keep tension bottled up and carry on working as if nothing is wrong, you are going to end up exploding like the fireworks at a fourth of July show.

Self-care can be as simple as taking some time to plan meals ahead of time so you aren't as stressed out later, or eating healthier so you feel better in the long run. Getting enough sleep is another one of the most important ways to take care of yourself. Often, it's something we overlook in our busy lives.

Socializing might not be among the first things to cross our minds when thinking about self-care because it involves other people.

However, having social contact can boost morale and prevent you from being isolated and feeling lonely.

Self-care can be both physical and mental. When you exercise, it can make a big positive impact on your life. So can meditation, which teeters between physical and mental. Changing the way you think is possibly the most challenging, yet most rewarding, way to have self-care.

So, take some time for yourself. If that means getting a massage and you have the means to do it, then by all means, do it! I know that can be time-consuming and possibly not on the cards for you, depending on your situation. So if that's the case, squeeze other things into your busy schedule that make you feel a little happier in your life. Read on for some ideas about how to do this.

CHAPTER 1

SELF-CARE MAKES YOU AN (EVEN MORE) AWESOME MOM

"Self-care is giving the world the best of you instead of what's left of you."
Katie Reed

Being a mother is demanding. However, it feels worth it when you watch your children grow in front of your eyes. It's the best feeling imaginable to see them laugh and smile, or feel their warm embrace when they snuggle into your arms. That's why you chose to be a mom, right? We're fed a rosy picture of life from a young age. Having a child and taking care of your family is part of what makes you a successful woman. But that rosy picture can conceal a lot.

You grow up believing that as long as you have a nice place to live, a loving partner who supports you, and happy children to care for, you should be content. Complaining about that is unreasonable and you should settle into doing what's expected of you. Am I right?

There's no doubt that when you're a parent, there will be sacrifices. *Many* sacrifices. You give and give and *give* until there's nothing left. I know—you're just trying to be the best mother and partner to your spouse/girlfriend/boyfriend, but don't forget to take care of yourself, too!

Society has it drilled into your brain that if you take time for yourself, you're being selfish. *What kind of mother would do that?* Well, why not? Why shouldn't you put yourself first sometimes? After all, you're a person, too! It's like there's an unwritten rule that once you become a mother, you aren't allowed to be your own person anymore.

No one asks how you're doing—it's always "How are the kids?" or "How's the baby?". Now that you're a mom, it can seem like you're only allowed to talk about your kids and dedicate your time to your family. What kind of crazy poppycock (love that word) is that?

No one puts these expectations on the dad. If he watches the children while you go to the store, he's "such a good father." Forget the fact that you've taken the kids to every doctor, dental, and optometrist appointment since birth. Or that you're the one who packs their lunches, makes dinner, buys their school clothes, washes their laundry, stays up with them all night when they're sick...you get the idea. Meanwhile, he takes them to the park one time of your many times, and he's the hero. It's okay—you can take a moment to scream into a pillow. I'll wait. Feel better now?

Motherhood is a thankless job, so why do we do it? Why do we give so much of ourselves with nothing in return? It's because we care. We care so much about everyone else's well-being that we neglect our own. Let's take one of my good friends Ellie for example.

Ellie is a 32-year-old wife of an IT executive and mother of two children, Bryce and Dallas, who are ages one and five. Ellie and her family recently moved to the East Coast, away from the life she knew. With no friends or family nearby, she's lost her support system.

Exhausted from the move, she pushes herself forward to deal with the needs of her family. As soon as they arrived at the new home, her husband instantly began working long hours to accommodate their now higher cost of living, leaving Ellie to handle everything on the home base alone. She suppresses the part of herself that feels out of place in this strange new town to unpack and make their house a home that her family will love.

Every morning it's the same: She wakes up before sunrise to prepare her husband's lunch for work. Then, she gets her older child ready for school while she feeds the younger child before dropping one off at school and the other at daycare. When she gets home, she gets to work on her chores—cleaning, picking up toys, mopping the floor, shopping for groceries, and everything else that keeps the house running smoothly.

Though her role is important, these routine, mundane tasks leave her feeling like she's leading an unfulfilling life. She's lost her sense of individuality and feels like she's not doing something she can really be proud of.

Let's face it, mopping the floor is not a satisfying job. It's an activity that's forced and makes her feel like she's imprisoned in the role of mother and stay-at-home parent. She has no time to reflect on those feelings because she's too exhausted. The time she's supposed to be sleeping is spent taking care of a crying baby. Someone has to do it. Her husband needs his sleep to wake up early and work to provide for the family. But what about Ellie? She works, too, even though she doesn't get an income or recognition for her work.

This has slowly led to an underlying resentment of her family. She loves them with all her heart, but sometimes she wonders if this is the right life for her. Why does she need to be the one to do everything? Why does she need to get up in the middle of the night when she works just as hard during the day? It makes her feel that because she's not the one making money, her work is less valuable, which is far from the truth.

Without Ellie making her husband's lunch and making sure he always has clean clothes to wear, he wouldn't be as successful with his career. Without her cleaning the home and making dinner for her family, they wouldn't have a home that makes them feel happy and safe. Ellie's self-sacrifice keeps her family going, even when they don't realize it.

In some ways Ellie is lucky she's a stay-at-home mom. For those of us who work, there are a lot of other factors; we try to fit everything in plus deal with the mom guilt that arises when we don't feel we're doing the best job for our family. Actually, I think all moms can relate to this feeling, whether they're a stay-at-home parent, a working parent, or a single parent.

When you think about it, books and movies often reinforce the idea of the self-sacrifice related to a mother's love. But this love stems from the mom doing something that enriches their child's life, like when a college student comes home and finally has a home-cooked meal and clean laundry. It gives the impression that a mom is only valuable when she is providing for her family. She's never respected simply for existing and being herself.

This idea is toxic to your image of yourself. When you're told something often enough, even subliminally, you believe it. So, what do you do? How do we change this subconscious image that's drilled into our brains?

Well, there are two things you need to do: First, you need to get rid of the idea that you're only a mom or a partner. Remember that you're an individual like everyone else is. Separate yourself from the idea of being a mom and a partner. I'm not saying to neglect your family and their needs, but understand that you're more than just that.

The second thing is to take care of yourself. There's a reason that flight attendants tell parents to put on their own oxygen mask before putting one on their child. As much as you want to put your children's well-being first, your children depend on you, and you can't take care of them if you don't take care of yourself first.

TAKE CARE OF YOURSELF

So, what is self-care? When you hear about a mom taking care of themselves, the image that probably pops into your head is a woman who goes to the salon or gets a manicure. While that can well be a form of it, self-care is much more than that.

Self-care is taking time to care for yourself, giving your mind and body a break from the constant responsibilities of being a mother and partner. Self-care is connecting with yourself. It's "finding yourself" and doing things that make you happy. You need to build a relationship with yourself, listen to your body's needs, and clear your mind from all that pent-up stress. When you do that, you can achieve a balance where you can take care of others while meeting your own needs. It might sound crazy, but self-care requires you to be a little selfish. And that's completely okay.

So, how do you achieve this balance?

Most people assume that taking care of yourself means eating healthy food, exercising, and getting enough sleep. While doing that is, of course, important, you also need something that reaches more than your physical being. Something that brings you joy.

What connects you to that joy? Is it art? Paint a picture. Make a craft. Draw. Sculpt. Maybe music hits that part of your heart that makes you feel whole. Sing. Play an instrument. Listen to that song that gives you goosebumps. If you love to read, get lost in another world through a book. Fall in love with the characters and watch them grow. Feel the heat before a first kiss. Experience the pain of love and loss and adventure.

But, don't stop there. Finding a few moments where you can just be with yourself will work wonders on your stress levels.

If at all possible, take a relaxing bath without interruption. Imagine sliding into the warm, bubbly water without children slipping their fingers under the door or begging to let them come in and splash around with you. Take a solo walk around the block where you can breathe in the fresh air without looking around constantly to make sure your kids aren't running out in front of a car.

If you can find a little more time for yourself, get a massage. Take a class. Go for a coffee run and enjoy your coffee inside a cafe by yourself. Have a spa day or a girl's night out. Go to a bar or karaoke with your friends. Even taking the time to shave your legs without interruption can feel like a major accomplishment.

Then there's the spiritual side of your life. Finding just a few minutes every day where you can sit quietly and just breathe.

You know what's funny? As a child, you avoid naptime like it's the plague. When you're an adult, a nap is this unachievable, mythical thing that we long for but never get to have. Yet, it can be the perfect way to recharge. Who can't use a little more sleep?

CHAPTER TAKEAWAYS

- Motherhood is demanding and requires sacrifice, but you need to take time for yourself.
- Self-care helps you deal with negative emotions so you aren't as exhausted and stressed out.
- Find something that brings you joy.
- Discover what makes you feel complete spiritually, mentally, emotionally, and physically.

CHAPTER 2
SLEEP YOUR WAY TO BEING THE BEST MOM

"The best bridge between despair and hope is a good night's sleep." E. Joseph Cossman.

Sleep is one thing that you never realize how much you'll miss until you don't get it anymore. Moms know what it's like to go without sleep. Why else would the term "mombie" exist? It's because we're always sacrificing our sleep to get things done.

I'm sure you were told to "sleep when the baby sleeps," but that's easier said than done. Sure, you could take a nap—or you could finally clean the living room like you've been meaning to for the past week. You're always putting your own needs on the back burner to keep up with the hectic lifestyle of being a parent. It's admirable, for sure, but it can have a negative impact on your body and mind. That rest that you're pushing away is something you need.

Sleep is essential to function. How often do you think: "Well, I might only get five hours tonight, but I'll make it up tomorrow?" Then, tomorrow you're only getting six hours because, silly you, you thought you could catch up on it later. Before you know it, you're a crabby mess with more bags under her eyes than a metropolitan socialite has in her closet. You're snapping at your kids, your partner, your coworkers, and possibly that nice cashier at the store. I know, you're usually not this grumpy, but you haven't had a decent night's sleep since you were in your second trimester.

Is a lack of sleep really that bad? Yes, I'm afraid so. When you don't get enough sleep:

- You're snappy and irritable, too tired to keep the she-devil in her cage, so you let her run free (to your partner and children's dismay).
- Your memory disappears. Poof! It's gone AWOL. Why are you reading this book again?
- Everything requires so much effort. Even reading this chapter can be exhausting as you force yourself to stay awake (and not because it's boring).
- You might agree to something just to make life easier. You're just too tired to think it through and now your toddler has six cookies instead of the usual two, so they'll be bouncing off the walls in about ten minutes.
- You gain weight as most of us eat more when we're tired thanks to our messed up hormones telling us we're hungry when we shouldn't be. Please, I cannot stress enough that your body is *beautiful* whether you weigh 100, 200, or 300 pounds. But you don't want all your effort on that keto or Paleo diet to go to waste because you're missing out on some much-needed sleep.

WHY IS SLEEP SO IMPORTANT?

Think of your body like a cell phone. It performs many functions, both basic and advanced, that help with your daily tasks. However, no cell phone can go on forever. Eventually, it shuts off and needs to charge. Your body is the same way. You have many functions that you perform daily, but eventually, you need to recharge so you can perform those functions again later. You do that with sleep. Not only does it recharge your body and mind, it also clears out your cache, so to speak. You're getting rid of all those unnecessary "files" by clearing the waste and plaque produced by your brain. Sleep helps to organize memories and regulate emotions.

Sleep helps to repair almost every tissue in your body. Without it, you risk harming your:

- Blood pressure
- Immune system
- Breathing
- Appetite
- Hormones
- Cardiovascular health

Sleep doesn't sound so bad now, does it? I know you're thinking: *It's not like I want to go without sleep—I just don't know how to fit it in with everything else going on.* Don't fret. I'll help you come up with a solution so that tonight, you'll be getting the sleep you not only want but *deserve*.

HOW DO I GET A GOOD NIGHT'S SLEEP?

- **Set a regular bedtime and *stick to it*.** I know it's hard. Honestly, sticking to a bedtime routine is hard enough for your child. And now I'm asking you to do it as well? Trust me, it can work. Forget binging on Netflix tonight. "Just one more episode" can wait until the weekend. Tonight, focus on going to sleep at a time that will allow you to get a decent amount of sleep.
- **Mind the "nana naps."** You know how if your toddler takes a nap after a certain time, they'll be up all night? Well, they aren't the only ones. A short power nap can help us get through the day when we're losing sleep at night. But be mindful of napping too long or too late in the day. If you have a baby that keeps you up all night and napping during the day is the only time to get some rest, by all means, go for it! But if your children go to sleep and wake up on a

traditional schedule, then try to avoid late-afternoon naps unless you really need one.

- **Increase your activity.** Everyone's heard someone say, "They'll sleep good tonight" when the kids are running around at a barbeque or birthday party. They wear themselves out and then crash. The concept is the same for adults. Add a little activity to tire you out. An evening stroll around the block after dinner or a jog in the morning are good ways to add a little exercise and ensure you'll fall asleep on time. Getting out in daylight is a good idea in the morning as that sets your body clock up to rest better later.
- **Manage your stress levels.** Stress is a major candidate for disruptive sleep. Whether it's lying awake for hours because you're too concerned with various problems, or waking up in the middle of the night from worry, stress inhibits your sleep. We'll go over stress management in a few chapters, but for now, remember that stress means poor sleep.
- **Cut back on caffeine.** After a certain time, trade the coffee for a lavender or chamomile tea. Usually, 2 pm is a good time to stop any caffeine intake. And if you know that drinking soda after dinner will keep you awake, skip it. Actually please skip the soda as it isn't a good idea any time (see chapter six).
- **Get enough sleep.** This probably goes without saying, but try to get the recommended amount of sleep. Most people need about eight hours, give or take an hour, for a decent sleep. If it means waiting until tomorrow to wash the dishes or fold the laundry, then that's okay. You aren't a superwoman, and, despite what society tries to tell you, you don't need to be. The world will not end if you wait until tomorrow to wipe down the stovetop.

CREATE THE OPTIMUM SLEEP ENVIRONMENT

Besides all these other steps, you can create an environment that will help your sleep.

- **Keep it dark**. If streetlights or morning sunlight are issues, get blackout curtains. Close the door so the hall light or nightlight doesn't shine in your eyes. Alternatively, wear an eye mask.
- **Face the clock away from you.** If you use a digital clock, turn it away so the light doesn't distract you and you end up worrying about the time. *It's midnight already? Oh no, I should be asleep.* Now you can't sleep because you're too concerned with the fact that you should already be sleeping. Just turn the clock to face away and put it out of your mind (and your eyes).
- **Turn your phone off.** If you use your phone as your alarm, then put the notifications on silent. There's no need to be in the middle of a deep sleep, only to be woken up by that group text from your friends without kids who stay up half the night. Who cares about that comment on Facebook or Instagram? It'll be waiting for you in the morning.
- **Set the temperature.** You don't want the room to be so cold that you're shivering all night, but you don't want it to be so stuffy that you can't sleep, either. Set the temperature to a comfortable setting. This might take some adjustment if your partner prefers a fan and you don't, but I'm sure you can find a middle ground that leaves you both sleeping in comfort.
- **Eliminate the noise.** Try to make the room as quiet as possible. If you don't like complete silence, try using a noise machine. White noise or sounds of the ocean might put you to sleep. Maybe a little classical music might help, too. There's plenty of apps or devices that you can buy to help with this. They will also help mask external noise you can't control.
- **Avoid blue light before bed.** Blue light from screens like cell phones, laptops, or televisions can disrupt your sleep. Melatonin is a hormone that your body produces that tells you, *hey, it's time to sleep.* Blue light prevents melatonin production, leaving your body saying *time for sleep? I think?*

Maybe? It's suggested for both kids and adults to avoid screen time for at least one hour leading up to bedtime. If you need to use electronics, try using the night mode. This helps relieve some of the strain your eyes might experience. Another option is to wear a pair of those funky blue light blocking glasses in the evening. Google it!

- **Burn essential oils before bed.** Lavender, vetiver, chamomile, ylang-ylang, bergamot, and cedarwood are wonderful scents for relaxation and sleep. Use an electric oil burner rather than one with a naked flame in case you doze off while it's burning.
- **Take a bath.** I know it's not related to your sleep environment, but it's too good not to include. Take a nice, relaxing bath before bed if you can. A few drops of essential oils, Epsom salts or magnesium flakes (these contain magnesium chloride which is absorbed better) can do wonders!
- **Take a Magnesium Supplement.** On the topic of magnesium, this amazing mineral can help you relax and get ready for sleep. There are many forms of magnesium: magnesium citrate and magnesium glycinate are absorbed better than magnesium sulfate and magnesium chloride.

WATCH WHAT YOU EAT AND DRINK

Watching your diet can help with sleep, too. I'm not saying to cut out red meats and only drink soy milk. Instead, think of the timing and the amount of food intake before bed.

- **Avoid caffeine after a certain time.** We already went over this one earlier, so I won't say much more. Just try to avoid coffee, soda, and green or black tea after 2 pm.
- **Avoid large meals before bed.** Not only is this unhealthy and a factor in obesity, it keeps your body busy digesting food when it should be relaxing for sleep.
- **Don't go to bed hungry.** Don't eat too much, but don't eat

nothing, either. There's nothing more distracting than trying to sleep when your stomach is growling. It's crying *let me eat*, while you're crying *let me sleep*. Then, you end up getting out of bed for that midnight snack you were trying so hard to avoid. If you're hungry before bed, try eating a small snack. Something that's not filled with sugar and isn't super dense.

- **A hot drink before bed is good**. Many of us grew up having a nice hot chocolate before bed. While it's true that warm milk is comforting and can help us feel sleepy, it's often more of a psychological affect than any substance in the milk causing drowsiness. Milk contains tryptophan, which increases the feel good hormone serotonin. But you would have to drink a lot of milk for it to affect your sleep. Plus, the sugar in hot chocolate is likely to spike your blood sugar levels and have the opposite effect to making you sleepy.

An occasional warm milk (dairy or almond) before bedtime can be helpful, but a better alternative is herbal tea. Chamomile in particular will help you relax and you can find herbal teas in the supermarket that are specially formulated to help you sleep.

- **Take magnesium before bed.** As mentioned above, magnesium is great for calming your mind, relaxing your muscles, and promoting a restful sleep. It can also increase the GABA levels, which is a natural calming effect on your body's nervous system.
- **Drinking water is good.** However, be wary of drinking too much water too close to bed because you might wake in the middle of the night to use the bathroom. You know your bladder and if you can handle it.
- **Try a melatonin supplement.** As mentioned above, melatonin is the hormone that your body produces to make you feel sleepy. If you're having trouble getting to sleep, taking a Melatonin supplement can help ensure you get to sleep. You can buy it in different dosages but start with a small 1 mg dose as that may be all you need.

WEIGHTED BLANKETS

Described as a "giant hug," these have become popular recently because they calm your heart rate and breathing. This allows for a relaxing sleep and helps with anxiety or depression. They were originally developed to help people with autism, cerebral palsy, restless leg syndrome, and dementia, but are now used much more widely. If you decide to join the weighted blanket crowd, look for one that is 10% of your body weight.

My husband is an ex-soccer player who was also a restless sleeper. While he was in dreamland, he would often act out, scoring his winning goals in his sleep and kicking me awake. While I was thankful he wasn't a semi-professional boxer, my sleep was suffering. In desperation, I ordered a weighted blanket online and am pleased to report that life transformed. Now my husband doesn't kick me throughout the night from his old glory days on the field. As a bonus, he says he also feels better rested in the morning.

SLEEP CYCLES

It's helpful if we now look at what sleep cycles are. While you sleep, your body goes through four stages.

1. **Non-REM Stage 1 Sleep**—This is when your muscles relax and everything slows down: your breathing, heartbeat, eye movements, and brain waves. This stage only lasts a few minutes.
2. **Non-REM Stage 2 Sleep**—Everything continues to slow, your body temperature drops, and your eye movements cease.
3. **Non-REM Stage 3 Sleep**—This is when you hit a deep sleep that lets you feel refreshed in the morning. Your brain waves are slow, your muscles are relaxed, and your breathing and heartbeat are at their lowest levels.
4. **REM Sleep**—This is the stage when you dream. Brain wave activity, heart rate, and blood pressure are all closer to the levels you experience when you're awake. Your breathing is

faster and more irregular, but your muscles are temporarily paralyzed, preventing you from acting out your dreams (well, most of the time–see above).

These sleep cycles take around 90 minutes per cycle. If you're getting a proper amount of sleep, you'll experience these cycles fully. However, if you have a sleeping disorder, like sleep apnea, you might not experience the deeper cycles, despite feeling like you're getting a decent sleep. Or, if you're a mom, your sleep cycles might be disturbed by your child standing by your bed at 3 A.M. giving you a heart attack. No matter how sweet they look during the day, it's never any less terrifying seeing them beside your bed at night, like the child from a horror movie.

SLEEP APNEA

This is a common sleep disorder. While it is most common in men over the age of 50 who are carrying some weight around their middle and neck area, it can affect anyone at any age. Even babies can suffer from sleep apnea. The worst part is that most sufferers are usually completely unaware they have it.

What causes sleep apnea? While you sleep, the muscles in your tongue and soft palate relax, causing you to snore as air passes in and out of your airway. With sleep apnea, these muscles relax too much and the airway will partially, or even fully, close up. Then, your brain says *hey we aren't getting enough oxygen—wake up!* Usually, you jolt awake enough to start breathing again, but not awake enough to realize what has just happened. This can happen hundreds of times each night, severely disrupting those precious sleep cycles we just talked about.

Though you might not be aware of it, anyone who's sleeping around you will be. You'll be snoring, and suddenly, they'll hear nothing but silence until you're gasping yourself awake. It can be alarming for those around you. Sleep apnea might be common, but if left untreated, it can be dangerous.

How do you tell if you have sleep apnea? Here's a few signs:

- Snoring
- Fatigue
- Low energy
- Difficulty with concentration
- Waking up with headaches
- Depression
- Frequent bathroom breaks throughout the night

If you believe you suffer from sleep apnea, schedule a visit with your doctor to get tested. These tests usually involve spending the night in a facility where they monitor your sleeping. Some sleep facilities can send you home with a monitoring device to screen for sleep apnea. This screening will at least give you an idea if your sleep is a problem.

As if moms don't have enough problems, they're more at risk of developing sleep apnea from the weight gain and hormonal changes caused by pregnancy. The problem is that many doctors still don't take sleep apnea as a serious health concern and don't screen for it. If you think you have sleep apnea, tell your doctor you want to be tested and don't take no for an answer. If the doctor you see tries to push it to the side, assuring you nothing is wrong, see another one. Ensure that you get the proper health care you deserve. I stress this because sleep apnea affects not only your sleep.

Sleep apnea can also lead to:

- High blood pressure
- Cardiovascular disease
- Obesity
- Migraines
- Diabetes
- Cancer
- Risk of accidents because of excessive sleepiness

Even if sleep apnea isn't the suspect, there are a number of other sleep disorders you can have. Remember my story above about my husband?

My husband suffers from REM Sleep Behavior Disorder, which is why he was playing soccer in his sleep (at my expense). During REM sleep, the brain can be just as active as when you're awake. Usually the body is paralyzed, so it doesn't act out those dreams. Just as well I hear you say. However, in my husband's case, his body wasn't cooperating and his limbs were not shutting off. Instead, they would flail about.

If you or anyone in your family is suffering from sleep problems, have it checked out. It could be something serious. Maybe it isn't, but if it is, it's better to find out and fix the issue before something bad happens. After all, sleep is vital. Sleep is your friend. You need it. Don't let your persistence to be the best mom outweigh your need for sleep.

CHAPTER TAKEAWAYS

- If you aren't getting enough sleep, you aren't able to live up to your fullest potential.
- You need sleep to recharge your brain and rest, so you can think straight and be a little less grouchy with your kids.
- Without enough sleep, you risk harming your health.
- Set a regular bedtime and stick to it. Like your kids, you need a regular bedtime, too. If you make it a routine, it will be easier to fall asleep at night. It's hard, but stick with it.
- Unless you really need it, forget the "nana" naps late in the day. These can prevent you from falling asleep when it's bedtime. It's like when your toddler has a late nap and doesn't want to go to bed at bedtime.
- Increase your activity. If you increase your physical activity during the day, it will make you tired later on, and falling asleep will be easier.
- Manage stress levels. Stress can keep you up at night. It can disrupt sleep and prevent sleep altogether. Make sure you aren't feeling too stressed if you want a decent sleep.
- Get enough sleep. Don't rely on functioning with only five hours of sleep every night. Make time to sleep more.

- Set up your environment for good sleep. That means it should be dark, quiet and not too warm.
- Avoid screens for at least an hour before bed. The blue light messes with your eyes and keeps you awake.
- Essential oils can help relax you. Try lavender, chamomile, or ylang ylang.
- Avoid large meals and caffeine. Avoid caffeine after 2 pm as it might keep you up late.
- Don't go to bed hungry. If you go to sleep hungry, you'll wake up with your stomach yelling at you, "why didn't you feed me?"
- Water before bed is fine but don't overdo it, so you're waking up to go to the bathroom.
- Try using magnesium before bed. It can help rest your mind and relax your body.
- Weighted blankets feel like a giant hug and can help you relax.
- Sleep apnea can lead to poor sleep and other health problems. See a doctor if you suspect you may have this issue.

CHAPTER 3
LOOK AFTER YOUR MIND (AND MAKE SURE IT LOOKS AFTER YOU)

"You can't always control what goes on outside, but you can always control what goes on inside." Wayne Dyer

What we think determines our perception of reality. What you think, you become. If you think negative thoughts, they manifest into other aspects of your life—your relationships with the people around you, for starters. That's why you need to take care of your mind, so it can take care of you. It's hard to force positive thinking when you're exhausted mentally, but it can make such a difference. Besides, stress will wear you out, too.

Your thoughts govern your emotions. This means that you have the power to determine what your reality looks like. You can decide what you feel and how you react. This is the most empowering thing you'll ever learn to do. When you learn how to control the way you see things, your life will change for the better.

Let's use Piper and Tracy as an example.

Both are struggling mothers who are exhausted and overwhelmed by their roles as mothers. In this example, their children ask for help with their homework. Between their careers and home life, both moms are strapped for time and feeling overworked.

Tracy's son asks her for help with his homework. She's in the middle of

cooking dinner, clearing the table, and trying to straighten up the kitchen at the same time. Tracy often tells herself her kids ask too much of her and they don't appreciate everything she does. Her reaction to her son asking for help with homework is to snap, telling him she doesn't have time to help him. She tells him that he's too demanding and needs to figure it out on his own.

Piper, on the other hand, takes the time to process what she's feeling. She, too, is trying to make dinner and fix the table while cleaning the kitchen. Instead of snapping at her child, she simply explains that mommy is busy at the moment, but if he can wait a little longer, she will help him after they finish eating dinner.

The difference between the two reactions is that Piper took a moment to think through things without blindly reacting. She understands that her children have demands that don't always fit into her tight schedule and it's not unfair for them to ask their mom for help. Taking a deep breath and processing the situation can help you decide whether you let the situation overpower you or if you take control and claim power over the situation.

OVERTHINKING

You remember that embarrassing thing you said to someone like five years ago? You think about what you could've said that was funny or less humiliating, but it doesn't matter because it already happened. The worst is when you think of a comeback after it's too late. Everyone is guilty of overthinking, though some of us do it more than we should.

Many moms find themselves in a downward spiral of overthinking. The problem with overthinking is that it stresses you out and makes you worry about things that you don't even need to worry about. It's healthy to think up a worst-case scenario, that way you prepare in case it happens. It's not healthy to dwell on the what-ifs to the point of suffering anxiety and depression. Quit over-analyzing everything.

Sure, moms worry, but sometimes we take it to a whole new level. There's no sense in beating ourselves up because our child had fast food for dinner. So what? They'll have twice as many carrots tomorrow. There, problem solved.

When you overthink, you obsess about something, whether past, present, or future. Those thoughts are set on repeat—a continuous loop playing over and over. When you're stuck in a loop, you get nowhere and make no progress. This keeps you from moving on. At its worst, overthinking keeps us stuck in the past or the future, taking us away from the present moment and what we should actually be focusing on.

Overthinking happens because of an unattainable, perfect ideal. It's exhausting trying to reach this unachievable idea of perfection. You're left feeling drained and vulnerable. If one small thing is out of place, everything will fall apart.

Controlling your mind is about accepting that the world is flawed and that you can't change it by thinking about it over and over again. It's not up to you how the world treats you, but it is completely your choice how you react to it. Once you see that the situation in front of you is unavoidable and you accept it, you won't feel so stressed out and be constantly overthinking things.

WHAT CAUSES OVERTHINKING?

According to Dr. Jeffrey Huttman, executive director of The Palm Beach Institute in Florida, overthinking "may include rumination, in which an individual is stuck mentally rehashing their past or present decisions and/or actions." He also states that overthinking can be traced to a lack of security because people who develop self-doubt and low self-esteem can't live without over-assessing everything that happens to them.

Moms feel self-doubt from the constant judgement they experience from society. No matter what you do, you often feel it's not enough. If you stay home with your children, you're seen as an oppressed woman from a traditional relationship where the woman belongs in the kitchen. If you decide to work, you're seen as neglectful and putting yourself before your children. There is no winning. This leads to over-thinking every decision you make, and who needs that?

Overthinking is often tied to anxiety, self-image, and people-pleasing. While there is a debate of whether it's biological or sociological—or nature versus nurture—it's safe to say that it's a genuine issue that needs to be taken seriously. By understanding where your over-thinking stems from, you can tackle it easier.

HOW TO STOP OVERTHINKING

Journaling

Writing in a journal is a tried and tested means for mental release. Why else do so many people have diaries? They need to get some of the mind clutter emptied out of their brain. Journaling has made a comeback recently, and many people have turned to two specific types of journaling to help with their stress.

The first type is to record your feelings. Purge your thoughts regularly: morning, night, or before a big event. This can help you realize your fears and anxieties.

While it's not necessary to look back on your entries, doing so can have its benefits. You might look back and realize that your worst-case scenarios were very different from how things actually played out. This is a humbling exercise that will reveal many of your fears to be completely unfounded. It will also teach you to approach your life more rationally.

Do you remember Ellie from chapter one? After moving to the East Coast, her fear was that she wouldn't make any new friends and that her relationship with her husband would change. However, through her journaling, she realized that her initial fears didn't happen. When she read her previous entries, everything she was worried about seemed so much smaller than they had before. Most of her fears proved unfounded.

The second type of journal is a gratitude journal. As an alternative to the first journal option, this one is based on positivity. Write what you feel grateful for. We often forget to acknowledge all the good things we have in our lives. Such a positive exercise can help you look beyond your worries and present a more wholesome and complete picture of your life.

Moms can forget just how wonderful their children can be, especially when they're stomping their feet and throwing themselves on the floor screaming because they didn't get to eat cookies for dinner. By writing down the small, adorable things they do every day, you'll be able to appreciate them more. Plus, you'll have these memories recorded, so when you look back, you'll think "wow, I forgot about that" and appreciate it all over again.

You can write in either type of journal, a combination of both, or with or without someone else. How you choose to do it is completely up to you. Try both and see what works best for you.

Create a Worry Schedule

In one study, researchers had individuals with anxiety disorders create a worry schedule, which meant that participants took half an hour every day to overthink and worry. This concept sounds crazy, but the study showed that those who had an overthinking period were less anxious and could get more sleep than those who did not.

Obviously, you can't limit your worrying to only thirty minutes a day, but creating a time slot for it allows you to focus your energy on it during the allotted time. It's the same concept as journaling. It gives you the chance to thought-dump everything out of your system at once. Then, when you feel the urge to worry and overthink throughout the day, you can postpone it until your "worry time." Chances are it may have become less worrisome by then too.

One problem with overthinking is that it hinders your progress to work and function, but postponing it allows you to continue with your work.

Thought Substitution

Whenever you feel you are descending into a spiral of bad thoughts, try to think about a completely different thing instead of trying to suppress the actual bad thought. The science is simple. If you are told not to think about purple trees, you will subconsciously think about purple trees. The more you try not to think about it, the more it will resurface in your mind. To stop thinking about purple trees, you need to think about blue flowers.

Another handy trick is to create multiple interpretations of the same event so that all your negative thoughts become less believable. If you have a terrible feeling about a certain day, try to think of two or three different ways in which it might go wrong. Now that you have created multiple variations of the future, you are free to treat them as products of your mind and not as actual truths.

If neither of those options work for you, try changing the way you word things to yourself. If you constantly tell yourself that you hate your life, change it up. Instead, say that you wish for a more fulfilling life. This gives the potential for change, rather than focusing on negative words like "hate."

LIVING IN THE PRESENT

I love this quote from Eckhart Tolle: "When you make the present moment, instead of past and future, the focal point of your life, your ability to enjoy what you do and with it the quality of your life increases dramatically."

Sorry to be the bearer of bad news, but the past is over and done with and we can never change it. The future is another land we haven't yet entered. Sure, we can plan for things so that the present is hopefully better, but we can't live from that future place.

Don't allow your mind to take you away from experiencing and enjoying the present moment. Sure, there will be moments you might wish you weren't experiencing, but they are all part of your life. You never get that moment back, so make the most of it.

CHAPTER TAKEAWAYS

- Journaling
- Try a thought-dump. Write about everything you're feeling to work through your fears.
- Try a gratitude journal. Every day, write down at least three things you're thankful for.
- Create a Worry Schedule and put aside a slot of time each day to worry.

- Change the Thought. If you're trying not to think of purple trees, instead think of blue flowers.
- Multiple Interpretations. If you're worried about an event, think of three ways it could end. It will make your initial fear seem less plausible.
- Change the Wording. Instead of saying "I hate my life", say "I wish my life were more fulfilling". This takes the edge off the negative thinking, replacing one thought with a less harmful one.

CHAPTER 4
KILL THE STRESS BEFORE IT KILLS YOU

"It's not stress that kills us; it is our reaction to it." Hans Selye

Being a mom is stressful. There's not enough time to do the million things you're expected to do. It's no wonder that so many moms are stressed beyond belief. And when you're stressed, it's not only you that suffers but your family, too.

Let me paint you a picture. I'm sure it will be easy to imagine.

You wake up after only five hours of sleep. You're already annoyed because you want to sleep in a little while longer but can't because if your child will be late to school again. You just know that the school will be too eager to send home a note that makes you feel like total garbage. Speaking of garbage, you forgot to take the trash down again, which means you missed trash pickup.

You force yourself out of bed and attempt to wake the kids. This is no easy feat because once again, they went to bed later than they were supposed to because they were up too late sneaking videos on their tablets.

When you finally do wake them up, you're rushing them to brush their teeth and get dressed. Of course, they take their sweet time. Are they *trying* to make you lose your mind? And where are their shoes? Why can't they ever just put their shoes on the shoe rack?

By the time you make it out the door, they've missed the bus, so you need to drive them in again. The entire ride to school is nothing but you yelling at them and telling them they need to stop being so irresponsible. Meanwhile, all you can think about is how badly you wish you had a cup of coffee.

Does this scenario make you feel stressed? Yeah, me too, and this is only the start. You haven't even begun the day yet.

It's understandable that you'd feel stressed; you have a lot on your plate. And I'm willing to bet that you've taken on the role of supermom with little help from anyone else. So, what do you do? How do you keep yourself from constantly feeling stressed out?

Before we talk about how you can get rid of your stress, let's talk about what happens when you feel stressed.

When you feel stress, your heart rate and blood pressure increases, which increases the levels of adrenaline and cortisol in your body, also known as the stress hormones. This is known as the fight-or-flight response. Basically, your brain is saying, "Something is wrong here and we need to fix it *now*." The fight-or-flight response is there for your survival, and because we usually think of survival as a life or death situation, it can make you feel stressed.

Obviously, when you feel stressed, it won't always be a life or death situation, but that doesn't stop the cortisol from kicking in.

So, now that you know the science behind the stress, let's figure out how to fix it.

RELIEVING STRESS

Write it Down

As mentioned in the previous chapter, writing in a journal can help with overthinking. It can also help you relieve stress because it's an outlet to release your negative emotions by sharing what you're thinking. Because it's a personal journal, you can be open and honest without the fear of judgement or ridicule. Clear your mind with a brain dump on paper. Write whatever you're feeling, what you're stressed about, or anything else you just want to get off your chest.

Gratitude journals have gained recent popularity because they are proven to transform your health, relationships, and quality of life. Simply write down what you're grateful for every day. It can be the people who surround you, having a roof over your head, clothes on your back, clean drinking water, or the friendly smile of a stranger. This will help you change your outlook on life in only a few months.

Exercise and Diet

As Elle Woods in *Legally Blonde* put it: "Exercise gives you endorphins. Endorphins make you happy. Happy people just don't shoot their husbands—they just don't." Exercise helps to give you mental clarity while having many physical benefits as well. I won't go into too many details because you'll see more of this in chapter seven. Just know that exercise can relieve stress by helping you mentally and physically.

For some people, starting with a diet is easier than exercising. You don't need to make drastic changes to lower your stress. Add some healthier food options while cutting back on some of the unhealthier ones (like sugar), and you'll see a major difference in your attitude.

Breathing and Mindfulness

Once again, I won't go into too much detail because we will cover breathing meditation and mindfulness in the next chapter. For now, we'll just brush through the topic and move on.

Have you ever heard the phrase "breathe through your belly?" When you take a deep breath, you should see your stomach raise while your chest remains flat. That's the proper way to breathe. Many people spend their time shallow breathing, meaning they breathe in through their chest and not their stomach. Breathing through your belly allows the air to flow into your lungs better and is better for meditation.

You can practice breathing deep anywhere: sitting at a stoplight, in a meeting, or waiting for the bus. Breathe deep and slow, and you'll improve your sense of calm.

Mindfulness goes hand in hand with breathing and meditation. All you need to do is be aware of the present moment without judgement. The best part is that you don't need to take time from your busy schedule to do it. Simply pause and focus your attention on the activity you're currently doing and your surrounding environment. Focus on your senses. What do you hear, smell, and see? Is the air cool or warm? Soon, you'll feel a sense of calm descend over you. Practice this throughout the day when you're doing something routine.

Music

Music is a major stress reliever. Whether it's the tune that's soothing or the memory that stems from a certain song, you can find peace in it. Many people find that classical music is calming, but really it's based on your own preferences. What music do you like? You might find that you're calmer when listening to heavy metal and screaming, as ironic as that may sound. Just play some music in the background when you're stressed and let it wash over you, absorbing your emotions.

Visualization Therapy

There's more than one way to relieve stress through visualization. You might try more than one type before finding what works for you.

Try envisioning yourself in a place that brings you peace. Many people find tranquility in the ocean and beach or possibly the woods, near a lake or waterfall. Most likely, your vision will involve nature, but it's completely up to you to visualize the place that makes you happiest.

If visualizing a place doesn't do it for you, try a color. Colors have meanings, representations and can affect our emotions. Fast-food establishments often use a red and yellow color scheme to promote an appetite. They say not to paint a nursery yellow because it will make a baby cry. Think of a color that makes you feel calm. Most people lean toward blue or green shades because they're related to nature, which is calming. Red is often exciting and induces anger or passion. It's your mind, so only you know what colors make you feel calm.

If using your mind to visualize is hard, try creating a vision board. Most people use these boards to motivate them toward their goals, but instead of a goal-oriented board, try using things that make you happy. Paste pictures of places that make you feel calm, pictures of your family or friends, or even quotes that make you feel better when you're down. The thing that's great about vision boards is that it's personal. You choose what you use.

Acupressure

There are natural practices that have been around for thousands of years that stand the test of time today. The ancient Chinese art of acupressure is one of them. It's similar to acupuncture and can be done at home without a qualified practitioner.

Acupressure functions on the principle that certain energies flow within your body. These energies get disturbed and blocked, leading to problems like stress.

There are two pressure points on your head. One is above your nose, between your eyes. The other is the soft spot on your head known as the crown. When you stimulate these two points with light pressure, energy is released, helping to remove the stress.

The key to acupressure is knowing the right points and placing the right amount of pressure.

Attitude is Everything

You can't control everything that happens in your life. You can, however, choose how you respond to it. Changing how you think is a good start to getting rid of your stress.

What you put into the universe is what you get back. If you think negative thoughts, you'll find negativity surrounding you. On the other hand, if you bring positivity into the world, that's what you'll get back. You'll find that the things you used to think about negatively, you can now put a positive spin on. Turn mistakes into learning experiences.

Drop the ideas or fantasies about how the people around you or the situations you're in *should* be. Things are as they are and you can't change other people and external circumstances. You can only change how you view them. Once you stop putting these expectations on people and the things around you, you'll find that you'll be a lot happier.

Talk About it

Most moms hold back on how they're feeling. They keep it bottled up to keep the peace. Unfortunately, this helps nothing. In fact, it often only leads to a bigger blow up.

If something is bothering you, just tell someone. Sometimes, having someone to vent to helps tremendously. If you don't have someone to talk with, speak with a counselor or helpline. There are free counselors available that you can find on Google and not every helpline is for emergencies. There are helplines for moms who just need a listening ear. The following are US-based organizations but for anyone not in the US, google to find ones local to you.

Helplines:

- *The National Parent Helpline*
- 1-855-4A-PARENT (1-855-427-2736)
- Available Monday through Friday, from 10 A.M. to 7 P.M., Pacific time
- *Parent Stress Line*
- 1-800-632-8188
- Available 24/7
- *Parenting Stress Helpline*
- 1-800-829-3777
- Available 24/7

If you don't feel comfortable talking over the phone, try an online support group.

Online support groups:

Motherly has a list of groups for moms and their families.

Blossoming Mothers Online Support Group is a support group where you can talk to other moms or professional counselors.

Baby Center offers groups and chats that are based on a number of parenting topics.

Facebook has groups of any type to choose from: for serious moms, silly and sarcastic moms, and even dads.

The Motherhood Center offers groups for moms who struggle with postpartum depression. They even have groups for dads.

Don't bottle up your emotions. Let them flow freely and you'll feel such relief.

Essential Oils

Everyone's heard of essential oils. They are powerful mood enhancers. You can add them to a diffuser or use them in a roller bottle. Different scents have different effects. Here are a few of the popular calming scents:

- Lavender
- Lemon
- Bergamot
- Chamomile
- Peppermint
- Ylang ylang
- Rosemary
- Sandalwood
- Geranium

Roller bottles are great for carrying around so you can stop and smell the calm whenever you need. You can buy little 10 ml roller bottles on Amazon and simply fill one with a carrier oil like liquid coconut, sweet almond, or jojoba. Then, add six drops of essential oil and gently tip the bottle a few times to mix. When you're stressed or feeling anxious, roll some onto the palms of your hands and take a few deep breaths. You can also roll the blend onto the pulse points on your wrists, behind your ears, or at the bottom of your throat—basically anywhere you would put your perfume.

Yoga or Tai Chi

Yoga is a mind-body-spirit practice that combines physical movement with breathing and meditation. A yoga session can leave you feeling calm, peaceful, and energized.

Similarly, tai chi is an ancient Chinese practice that combines flowing movement with breathing and mindfulness. It's a form of moving meditation that promotes harmony and health and is a great way to relieve stress.

The good news is just about anyone can do yoga and tai chi. There are different styles of both practices, so you can look around and find one that resonates with you. These days there are numerous websites where you can find classes so you don't need to leave the house.

Laughter

Laughter is the best natural medicine for stress. You might feel weighed down by life. There's a thousand things to do and not enough time, so it makes sense that fun isn't a top priority on the list. Sometimes, you need to make the time to have a little fun and laugh. The way we see ourselves and our situations can drastically change when we look at it with a lighter heart. Circumstances appear different when you're happy and carefree.

I know it's hard to find time for fun when you're so busy. Why not blend the two together? When you're cooking dinner, listen to a stand-up comedy act. Watch a funny movie when you're folding clothes. Are you scrubbing the bathroom? Put a funny show on your phone and watch it while you clean. It's an instant stress-buster.

Go Outside

Nature has a way of healing and calming us. It's the perfect place to practice mindfulness, but it's also the best place to try grounding—also known as earthing.

When you're grounded, you feel stronger, more resilient, and centered. You'll also notice your stress and anxiety levels reduce, your digestion improves, your immune system is stronger, and you're getting better sleep. These are only a few of the reported benefits of grounding.

All you need to do is go outside and touch the earth. Walk barefoot in the grass or dirt. Lie on your back and soak up the essence of the world. You're connecting with the earth on the most basic level. While you're doing this, the earth's natural electric charge stabilizes your physical body.

SUPPLEMENTS FOR STRESS RELIEF

Giving your body the right fuel is more important than ever if you're under stress. In a catch-22 situation, your body will use up key nutrients faster when you're stressed—which can then make you more prone to stress.

A healthy, balanced diet will help, but it's often not high on the priority list at these times. Many of us reach for the alcohol, chocolate when life gets tough.

Luckily, there are natural supplements to help you deal with stress. If you can, consult a natural health practitioner. They can give you tailored advice that matches your individual needs.

The right supplements will help:

- Relieve stress
- Keep up your body's immune defences strong
- Improve your ability to cope.

Magnesium

Magnesium is crucial to our health and wellness. It's used in over 300 biochemical reactions in the body, including:

- Energy production
- Even blood sugar levels
- Blood pressure regulation
- Protein production

Many people are deficient in magnesium. Caffeine and alcohol can increase the loss of magnesium through frequent urination. Not to mention, stress can use it up faster, too, which is ironic considering it's important for relieving stress and anxiety, relaxing your muscles, calming your mind, and promoting a restful sleep.

If you choose a Magnesium supplement, the recommended daily dose is 300-400 mg[2].

Options for increasing your levels of magnesium include:

- Take a supplement: Magnesium glycinate is the best-absorbed magnesium supplement. Its high bioavailability means your body can use it more easily. It's also less likely to cause diarrhea and nausea, which can happen with some cheaper forms of magnesium supplements.
- Apply it topically: Your skin can absorb magnesium so it acts faster than an oral supplement. Magnesium oil or magnesium cream are simple to use—though the oil can sometimes irritate to your skin.
- Add it to your bath: This is a great way to enjoy the benefits of both the magnesium and the whole bath experience. Traditional Epsom salts contain magnesium sulfate and are a cost effective form of magnesium. Alternatively, magnesium chloride flakes have a more easily absorbed form of magnesium that your body can use more readily.
- Add more to your diet: Foods rich in magnesium include

bananas, oily fish, dark leafy greens such as spinach, kale, swiss chard and beet greens, brazil nuts, cashew nuts, avocado and dark chocolate (yay!).

B Complex Vitamins

B vitamins are involved in energy production and keeping the body functioning properly. They help your body make neurotransmitters, which improve your ability to handle stress. You don't need to know all the ins and outs of B vitamins, but for those of you that love the details, here they are.

Vitamin B6 (Pyridoxine) is used to make neurotransmitters (chemical messengers) called serotonin and GABA. Stress and anxiety deplete both these neurotransmitters. This makes B6 particularly important to help relieve stress. The recommended daily dose for women is 1.6 mg and for men is 2 mg.

Vitamin B5 (Pantothenic Acid) reduces the amount of cortisol production caused by stress. This takes the load off the adrenal glands and improves ability to cope with stress. The recommended daily dose for adults is 4-7 mg.

Vitamin B9, (Folic Acid/Folate), is also another B vitamin important for mood. Folate deficiency is linked to a range of health problems, including major depressive disorder. The recommended daily dose for adults is 400 micrograms.

Vitamin B12 (Cobalamin) deficiency has a profound effect on mental health and wellbeing and the ability to cope with stress and anxiety. Unfortunately, B12 deficiencies are common. If you're a vegetarian, vegan or elderly, you may be more susceptible to low B12 levels. Some people don't absorb B12 well, which also results in a deficiency. The recommended daily dose for adults is 2 micrograms.

If you notice any of the following B12 deficiency symptoms, check with your health practitioner:

- Weakness
- Fatigue

- Anaemia
- Foggy brain and/or memory loss
- Numbness or tingling in your hands, legs, or feet.

Vitamin C

As well as being important for your immune system, Vitamin C helps reduce the physical and psychological effects of stress. This crucial vitamin regulates blood pressure and production of cortisol and plays an important role in managing stress.

Take a good supplement twice per day to help you through stressful periods. The recommended daily dose for adults is 75-125 mg though you can take up to 2000 mg for boosting your immune system if it's required[2]. It's better to take two smaller doses rather than one large dose. Vitamin C is a water soluble vitamin and your body will simply excrete what it doesn't use.

Taurine

Taurine is an amino acid that has a role in regulating mood and stress and has an anti-anxiety effect on the central nervous system. Your body uses taurine to make GABA (gamma-amino-butyric acid). GABA is the main calming neurotransmitter that turns stress hormones off.

Chromium

Chromium is a mineral that helps to stabilize blood sugar and can help with maintaining healthy moods and may help to regulate cortisol levels. The recommended daily dose for adults is 50-200 micrograms.

Zinc

Zinc is also important for your immune system. There are hundreds of reactions in your body involving zinc.

Many people are deficient in zinc, as the levels in the soil these days are low and your body doesn't store it. Zinc deficiency affects your digestion and nutrient absorption, making you less able to cope with stress. The recommended daily dose for adults is 15 mg or 0.2 mg per kg of body weight[2].

Essential Fatty Acids (EFAs)

Essential fatty acids have a protective effect on the brain during chronic stress and are shown to reduce anxiety. The reason they are called "essential" is you have to get them from your diet as your body can't make them.

Even if you're not stressed, EFAs are highly recommended. The main EFAs that are essential to our diet are:

Omega-3s

These EFAs are an important part of the body's cells. They are anti-inflammatory and promote:

- Heart health
- Mental health
- Brain development
- Reducing the inflammation that contributes to a range of diseases

Omega-6s

These are also essential, as we use them for energy. However, the Western diet has an unhealthy, very high level of omega-6s which promotes inflammation.

Studies show that large amounts of omega-6 fatty acids and a high ratio of omega-6 to omega-3 ratio leads to diseases such as:

- Cardiovascular disease
- Cancer

- Autoimmune and other inflammatory diseases.

The recommended ratio of omega-6 to omega-3 EFAs is 4:1 or even less. The problem is, our diets often have ratios of 10:1 or even higher.

So basically, you don't want to be supplementing with omega-6 EFAs, but you definitely want to increase your intake of omega-3.

There are many forms of omega-3s with the most common supplement forms being EPA (eicosapentaenoic acid) and DHA (docosahexaenoic acid). The recommended daily dose of DHA/EPA for adults is 1-3 mg[2].

Herbal Support

There are many herbs that can help relieve stress:

- Ginseng, Rhodiola and Rehmannia support the adrenal glands, improving stress resilience and increasing a sense of wellbeing.
- Gingko reduces cortisol levels
- Withania reduces anxiety and tension

Other herbs that have a relaxing effect include valerian, kava, chamomile, hops and passionflower. Again, it's well worth consulting a health practitioner, so you get supplements that are recommended for your personal situation.

FOODS TO AVOID WHEN YOU'RE STRESSED

Alcohol

OK, this is a potentially sensitive subject. Who doesn't love a glass of something to help take the edge off what's happening and help us relax? Most of us believe alcohol calms us down and it does—in the short term.

However, in the long run, alcohol increases anxiety and depression, making it harder to deal with stress. The effect of alcohol is to increase the adrenal hormones, adrenaline, and cortisol. This interferes with normal brain chemistry and sleep cycles, so is best avoided in times of great stress, anxiety or insomnia.

Refined Carbohydrates

Under stress, it's all too easy to reach for convenience foods. Or assure ourselves that eating chocolate or ice-cream will help. This is probably the worst thing we can do to ourselves.

Sugar and white flour play havoc with blood sugar levels as they are high GI (glycemic index) foods. Shortly after eating high GI foods, sugar is released into your bloodstream, causing a fast spike in blood sugar levels. In response, your body releases insulin to clear the sugar from the bloodstream and move it into storage for later use.

This quick response causes blood sugar levels to plummet. After around an hour, you may feel low on energy, irritable or even aggressive—and hungry again. Try eliminating refined carbohydrates from your diet for three weeks and notice how different you feel.

Caffeine?

"Nooo" I hear you say. "I absolutely cannot cope without my morning hit." Don't worry, it isn't necessarily bad. On the one hand, caffeine raises cortisol levels in your body. If you're already anxious or stressed, your cortisol levels are likely to be high and caffeine may well make you feel a lot worse.

On the other hand, coffee consumption is linked to elevated mood and even reduced levels of depression. So this is clearly a personal one and you will need to decide for yourself whether to keep drinking coffee. If it's making you feel anxious, or affecting your sleep, then it's time to find an alternative drink.

DIGITAL DETOX, SELF-LOVE AND REACHING OUT

Digital Detox

Social media is both a blessing and a curse. It gives us the opportunity to connect with friends, family, and even strangers. Unfortunately, it also means that the annoying girl from high school can send you friend requests and ask you to join her pyramid scheme for selling those even more annoying weight-loss beverages.

While social media has its fun moments, it has its negative ones, too. All this connection to the world can leave you overstimulated and stressed out. When that happens, do a digital detox. Cleanse yourself from social media by taking a break from everyone else's life and focusing on your own.

Self-Love

We're often led to believe that in order to love ourselves, we need validation from outside sources. But you don't need a man, boss, coworker, or anyone else to make you feel deserving of love and acceptance. You just don't!

You were born unique, , and completely loveable. Nothing anyone else says or does can ever change that. Many of us have a hard time believing that, but trust me, it's 100% true.

Practice self-love. Once you feel confident in yourself, you'll feel confident about tackling everything the world throws your way.

Reaching Out

Sometimes, you need support from others to deal with your struggles. Don't be afraid to reach out! You can find solace in a support group or a social group with other moms who are dealing with issues similar to your own.

Contact a therapist if you don't feel comfortable talking to a friend or family member. There are plenty of hotlines that are non-emergency. There are even hotlines for moms who just need a listening ear. If you're interested in this, check out the hotlines mentioned earlier in this chapter.

However you decide to reach out, just know that you *aren't alone* and there's *no shame* in asking for help. No one comes out of this world doing everything completely on their own. No one.

CHAPTER TAKEAWAYS

- Exercise releases endorphins, which makes you happy.
- Focus on your breathing and use mindfulness to relax your mind.
- Music is filled with emotion. Use it to enhance your feelings.
- Visualize a place or color that makes you feel relaxed and at peace.
- Vision Boards can have an assortment of images you see daily to remind you of the things that make you feel less stressed.
- Acupressure. Knowing what parts of your body to apply light pressure can help relieve your stress.
- Attitude is everything. Think positive and you will feel positive.
- Talk about it. If something is bothering you, or you feel stressed and/or depressed, talk about it. If you don't feel comfortable talking to your family and can't afford a therapist, call a helpline or join an online forum support group made for parents.
- Gratitude journals can help you appreciate your life. You'll focus on what you're happy with.
- In contrast, writing about your problems can help you work through them.
- Certain scents can make you feel calm. You can put essential oils in a diffuser or on a roller to roll on your skin directly.
- Yoga and Tai Chi are two physical practices that help you clear your mind and move your body in ways that release the tension.
- Laughter really is the best medicine. Listen to a stand-up

comedian while making dinner, or watch a comedy. Let yourself laugh.
- Go outside. Being outside is relaxing because you're reconnecting with the Earth.
- Try magnesium; Take a supplement, add it to a bath, or add more to your diet.
- A digital detox will work wonders on your mental health.
- Love yourself.

CHAPTER 5
BREATHE YOUR WAY TO SANITY

"Be the master of mind rather than mastered by mind." Zen proverb

I've said it before, and I'll say it again: Being a mom is overwhelming. Sometimes, you lose your cool. Between work, school, a messy house, homework, doctor appointments, cooking dinner, laundry, and everything else, it can seem like the world is trying to swallow you whole. How are you expected to keep up with it all?

STILL YOUR MIND

You may have heard of meditation. You might have even tried it, too. There are so many benefits to your mental state. Meditation can help your physical state too.

Still my mind? How can I do that when there's so much running through my mind? I know it can seem impossible when you have no free time, but I swear, it *is* possible! Maybe it would help if I told you the story of Louisa, a mother of two young children.

Louisa always wanted to have kids. Squishy cheeks and cozy snuggles were all she could think about when she was pregnant. She had no idea life would be that chaotic when she had her first child. Then, the second one came

along two years later and she was stressed to the max. She constantly told herself that something needed to change but wasn't sure what to do. So she continued her daily routine in the hope that somewhere along the line things would get better.

One day, she was cleaning the living room, as she always did. She left the room for a few minutes to straighten the bathroom, and when she came back, the living room was trashed again. Toys were everywhere. Melted chocolate was smeared all over the couch and television. She was only gone for ten minutes! How could they destroy the living room to that degree in only ten minutes? It looked like a tornado had been through there, right after she just cleaned it.

That was it. That was the point that made her completely blow up. We're talking about a Mount Vesuvius blow up, and her kids were Pompeii waiting to happen. She yelled so loud that the neighbors didn't look her in the eyes for two weeks. Yeah, that was her breaking point.

She realized that if she wanted a change; she needed to make it herself. She spoke with her oldest child's counselor and asked for tips on how she could keep calm when she's ready to blow. The counselor suggested mindfulness and meditation. After discussing a few ways to do this, gave it a try. What'd she have to lose?

It took a few different techniques to find what worked for her, which was blending a few into one. It's helped tremendously, too. Last week, she walked into the bathroom to get the girls out of the bath, and the floor was covered in water from the splashing they promised they wouldn't do. There was soap on the toilet, and they had emptied the rest of their bubble wash in the tub. It was a mess. A mess that, had it happened before she discovered meditation and mindfulness, would've made her flip her lid.

However, she knew how to handle this without yelling. She wrapped the girls in their towels and sent them to their room to put on their jammies, and then she walked out of the bathroom to her "cozy corner." That's what she calls her special calming place. Taking a seat, she counted to ten, taking a deep breath between each number, and then she visualized the beach. The gentle breeze against her skin. The blue water that blends into white waves rushing over the soft, yet gritty, sand. And the smell. Oh, the smell—you wouldn't think salty smells so good, but it does.

Once she felt calm enough to pull herself away, she could handle whatever was thrown her way. Instead of yelling at her kids, she went to their room and explained that they broke their promise not to get water on the floor and they were going to help her clean it up.

Using mindfulness and meditation has allowed Louisa to gain control of her outbursts and how she reacts when her children misbehave. It's transformed her life because now when she gets mad, she doesn't yell. Instead, she takes a moment to calm herself by daydreaming of the calming beach waters. Meditation and mindfulness have changed her entire mindset.

CALM YOUR NERVOUS SYSTEM

One easy way to quickly calm your nervous system is to breathe in counting to four, hold the breath for a moment, then breathe out counting to eight. Actually, it can be any number but the important thing is that the out-breath takes twice as long as the in-breath. This sends a signal to your nervous system to relax. This is a very useful tool as you can do it anywhere, at any time. And nobody will know you're doing it! Go ahead and try it right now and see how you feel.

Another technique, used by Navy SEALs to stay calm, is called box breathing. The technique is a powerful stress reliever and helps heighten concentration and performance. As the name suggests, the technique is like the four sides of a square.

To practice box breathing, sit comfortably with a straight spine and do the following:

1. Breathe in slowly and steadily through your nose for the count of four.
2. Hold the breath for the count of four.
3. Breathe out slowly and steadily through your mouth while counting to four.
4. Hold with your breath out for the count of four before repeating the entire process several times.

MINDFULNESS

Mindfulness is a state of awareness. When you are mindful, your mind, heart, and soul are fully focused on the present moment. You accept your feelings without judgement. You observe and understand your feelings without thinking if they are right or wrong. You're viewing these thoughts deliberately from a distance and with complete objectivity.

When you are mindful, you are aware of your surrounding environment and the thoughts, feelings, and sensations felt by your body. You are aware only of the present moment. Forget looking to the past or worrying about what your future holds. Focus only on the present and live in that moment.

The Science Behind It

Now, let's get to the scientific aspect. Research shows immunity and brain function are positively affected by mindfulness meditation. Your immune system is boosted while your level of stress is reduced and your mind is restored.

Separate research from 1999, 2002, and 2006 suggests that mindfulness increases metacognitive awareness. I know I'm throwing around some big words now. Let me explain. When you practice mindfulness, you're aware of your thoughts and feelings, but view them as passing and not as a reality. You're aware of how you think and understand the why and how behind it, without setting these thoughts in stone. Basically, you can evaluate your own thoughts without getting too tied up in them.

Mindfulness also changes the physical density of your brain in areas related to kindness, memory, learning, and feeling. It helps you remember more and remain attentive longer.

Mindfulness can affect you positively by reducing:

- Stress
- Anxiety
- Fear

- Anger

It's linked to higher levels of:

- Satisfaction
- Conscientiousness
- Self-esteem
- Empathy
- Autonomy
- Competence
- Optimism
- Happiness

Studies have shown that by not practicing mindfulness, you can experience negative traits like:

- Depression
- Dissociation
- Emotional instability
- Stress
- Anxiety

Mindfulness is a great tool for depression. I'm not saying to throw your antidepressants in the toilet and flush them. Don't do that. Ever. I'm saying that with enough practice, it can help alleviate your depression as an addition to medicine. Always consult your doctor before making any decisions relating to depression medication.

Practicing Mindfulness

Being conscious and being mindful are two different things. Everyone wakes up in the morning, conscious of what's going on around them. In a sense, reality is just an illusion. Still confused? Let me give you an example: your house is a wreck today. Usually, this might send you into a fit of anxiety to get the house clean in time for supper. Mindfulness will tell you that material possessions and cleanliness are merely illusions to begin with. The cleanliness of your house does not determine who you are as a person. It doesn't make you any less loving toward your children or partner. I'm not saying to let the mold grow and leave trash lying around, but don't stress yourself over something that is simply cosmetic.

Find a place that makes you feel at peace. Let's look at Alex, who used mindfulness to help overcome her depression.

Alex was living with an illness that was slowly taking over her life and not in a physical way. She was feeling self-pity and loathing that was gradually pushing her friends away. She didn't have many friends to begin with, so pushing away those she spent time with was taking a toll on her mental state.

At the top of a nearby hill was a small church that was no longer in service. One day, when she was struggling harder than usual, she took a walk up the hill to the church. She had no idea what she was looking for in this walk. Maybe just peace of mind or something to bring her clarity. Either way, she found it.

The view was stunning. She could see the colors of the world around her bursting to life: the patchwork of autumn leaves covering the trees and the ground surrounding them; the sunlight twinkling off the stream that wraps around the bottom of the hill; and even the crisp, fresh air hugging her face as she watched the bustling town life below.

What she saw made her feel small in the world, but not in the sense that she was insignificant. Instead, she felt like a part of something greater as she watched the orange and yellow hues of the sun in the clouds slowly turn to a darker shade of red and purple as the sun set. For a moment, she felt close to God.

It doesn't matter if you are religious or not. Mindfulness brings out a sense of spirituality and being one with your surroundings. Some people find this at the beach, a waterfall, the park, or any other place of nature. Not that nature is the only place you can be mindful. You just need to be somewhere that you can put everything into perspective and feel at peace.

When you find your place of grounding, you can use mindfulness to make yourself aware of the moment you are in, rather than the future or the past. Mindfulness dismisses the past and future because one has gone and the other has not yet arrived. The only point in time you have is the present.

MEDITATION

You can enhance your mindfulness through meditation. Meditation is the practice of focused concentration. It has many benefits, both physically and mentally, such as increased focus and concentration, reduced depression and anxiety, lowered blood pressure, and decreased likelihood of heart disease and chronic pain. There are different ways to meditate. Before we get into some of the different techniques, let's go over the basic how-to.

How-To

1. Sit in a position that straightens your back so the energy can flow freely.
2. Close your eyes and relax your muscles.
3. Breathe in slowly through your nose. Allow your lungs to fill with air until full.
4. Hold that breath for a moment before releasing it slowly.
5. Let your mind clear. When you notice your thoughts drifting, pull it back to focus on your breathing.
6. Continue doing this until you feel relaxed.

While many people will do this for about half an hour, it is totally fine to do it for shorter periods of time. There are many types of meditation in which these steps vary. For instance, you might keep your eyes open and focus solely on an object in front of you. The object is usually something that promotes peaceful thinking, like a flower or a statue of Buddha. Maybe instead of sitting in position, you choose to walk instead. The idea is to concentrate on something to clear your mind, free of distractions. Let's look at a few other techniques for meditation.

Body Scan Meditation

1. Sit or lie down in a comfortable position.
2. Steady your breathing as you did above.
3. Bring your attention to the sensations of your body. Focus on specific parts of your body. Start with your toes and move up to your feet, ankles, thighs, and so on, moving up to your hands and fingers, wrists, shoulders, neck, and face until you reach the top of your head.

This is similar to ancient meditation techniques practiced by monks to unblock the flow of energy throughout the body. By clearing your chakras, or pools of energy within your body, you're allowing your mind to access a higher state of calm and clarity.

We don't always realize how much stress affects us physically. By straightening your shoulders, stretching your limbs, unclenching the tension in your fists, you can experience a relief from your stress and anxiety. Practicing this type of meditation will allow you to respond to stress by relaxing your body and feeling the sensations of it naturally. This can slow or stop the process of your spiraling thoughts. You'll also be able to identify which parts of your body hold the most tension.

Relaxation Breathing

1. Relax your body.
2. Close your eyes.
3. Breathe in slowly while counting to four. Imagine the oxygen flowing through your nostrils and into your lungs.
4. Hold that breath and count to four.
5. Exhale while counting to eight. As you release your breath, imagine all the stress and insecurities leaving with it.
6. Repeat these steps until you feel relaxed.

The point of this short meditation technique is to give you a break from the stress so you can just... breathe. It's not a technique to help you process your problems, but to just take a break from them. While you're doing this, try to clear your mind from external thoughts and issues. Block out the sensory and emotional stimuli.

This technique is popular because it's an instant relief for moments of anxiety. It's quick and can be done anywhere, which is a bonus for your busy schedule. Plus, it helps to regulate your heart rate and blood pressure instantly.

When you exhale for a longer period than you inhale, your brain signals your fight-or-flight response (which is responsible for stress) to calm and relax. By relaxing, you're able to handle your stress logically and less impulsively.

Breathing Meditation

1. Sit up straight and relax your body and muscles.
2. Breathe in and out, slowly counting each breath. (Inhale one, exhale one. Inhale, two, exhale two... etc.)
3. Count up to ten and then repeat the cycle five more times.
4. While you're breathing, imagine the breath flowing throughout your body like you would with relaxation breathing and then exhale the negativity.

After doing this for several minutes, your breathing will become calm and centered. The point behind this technique is to treat your brain like a muscle that needs to be exercised to function properly.

One study found that after two months of daily practice, MRI scans revealed an increase in the grey matter in the brain. Grey matter is good. It's rich in nerves and neurons relating to controlling your focus and anxiety and found in people with higher IQ scores.

Visualization Meditation

Remember Louisa, the mom above? She used visualization to calm herself when the kids made a mess in the bathroom. Visualization is using your mind to create an image that brings you peace. Maybe it's a single item, like a lily. It could be a place, like a beautiful mountain landscape with a waterfall cascading down the side, or, if you're like Louisa, you prefer to think of the beach. Picturing your family on a picnic, laughing while your children run around the lush, green grass might be the image that calms you. Whatever it is, you're going to close your eyes, focus your breathing, and imagine it. Don't forget to use your senses! What do you smell? Is it the musky smell of a fire or the floral scent of a flower? What do you hear? Can you taste anything? What about feeling? What sensations do you feel? You want to be completely absorbed in your magical place of peace.

MOVEMENT

What is movement meditation? You guessed it: movement. This can apply to so many things. The first thing that probably pops into your mind is yoga, right? We're talking about meditation and movement; the two go hand-in-hand. Well, yoga is a form of moving meditation, but it isn't the only one. Don't worry, I'll go into yoga a little more below, but for now, let's explore those other meditative movements.

Moving meditation is when you focus on the movement of your body and sensations you feel. You might not realize that you already do this.

When you're washing dishes, does your mind shut off for a bit, and you focus only on the warm water submerging your hands or the grimy soap scrubbing off bits of food? I know it's gross, but you don't care because, at that moment, you're only focused on one thing: washing the dishes.

If you like jogging, then you might focus on the way the pavement feels beneath your shoes or the cracking sound it makes against the asphalt. How about the way your chest heaves in and out with every breath?

Do you enjoy gardening? How about the way the dirt feels against your fingers or gloves? The smell of the earth is gratifying and grounding.

There are many ways to meditate while you're moving, and the best part is that you can do it while you're doing your regular chores.

Taking some time to clear your mind while also taking care of folding that laundry is a win-win—it's multitasking at its finest.

YOGA

You probably have a friend or relative who does yoga and tells you all about how it's made their life so much better. How? As opposed to regular exercise, yoga combines physical exertion with self-awareness and compassion. It emphasizes the connection between the body and the mind.

Practicing yoga trains your brain to become more tolerant of stress. It can regulate your heart rate and hormone levels and reduce your depression. The philosophy behind yoga is to be non-judgmental toward yourself and others, which is helpful because a lot of your stress emerges from being so hard on yourself.

You can use the breathing techniques above to enhance your yoga experience. When you combine breathing with mindfulness, yoga can really have its benefits. The best part is that you don't need to know every position with perfection. Knowing even a few poses will take you a long way.

The RAIN Method, promoted by Tara Brach, is a method that combines mindfulness and self-compassion. You can use it when you face a difficult situation by following four steps.

R- Recognize what is happening and how you are feeling.

A- Accept the feeling and allow things to happen as they do without judgement.

I- Investigate your inner responses with gentleness.

N- Natural awareness. Remind yourself to not identify with the emotion, state or experience. Tara Brach prefers the N of this step to stand for "nurture" and suggests you offer comfort to the part of you that is distressed.

Note from the author:

While this chapter provides information to get you started in meditation and mindfulness, I felt that this is such an important topic, I've written a book expanding on this topic. Aimed at all moms who really don't have time for a regular, full-on meditation practice, *Be a Mindful Mom* is due out later this year.

CHAPTER TAKEAWAYS

- Mindfulness is a state of awareness. You're focused on the present moment, without judgement.
- Mindfulness can affect you positively by reducing stress, anxiety, fear, anger, depression.
- It's linked to higher levels of satisfaction, conscientiousness, self-esteem, empathy, autonomy, competence, optimism, happiness.
- Practice mindfulness by taking a moment to focus on the present moment. Don't think about the negatives and don't focus on what you want to change. Only what is.
- Relax your body, sit in a comfortable position, close your eyes, focus on your breathing, and allow your mind to let go.
- Body scan: focus on the sensations of your body. How do different areas like toes, arms, face, etc. feel?
- Relaxation breathing: A breathing technique that allows you quick relief from stress and anxiety. This technique is to take a moment to literally breathe.
- Breathing meditation is like the above, only you're focusing on how the breathing feels. Imagine the breath going in deep and exhaling the negative energy pent up inside.
- Think of a place you'd like to be. Visualize it. Think of a person who makes you happy. Or a pet that makes you smile. The point is to focus on something visual that makes you feel calm.
- Focus on everyday movement to help clear your mind at the same time. Focus on your shoes hitting the pavement when you run, or the water rushing over your fingers when you wash dishes.
- Yoga is a great stress reliever that combines activity with mindfulness and breathing.

CHAPTER 6
EAT FOR YOUR LIFE

"Good news—food is a form of self-care!" Anon

Sorry folks, let me just tweak that above quote. It should read "The right food is a form of self-care". Let's have a look at what that is.

The world seems to have gone food and diet mad lately. Which is great news in that people are becoming more aware of how important healthy eating and putting quality fuel into our bodies is. A healthy diet determines not just our physical health, it also affects our mental health and how we feel.

But you may not want to lose weight or introduce keto, paleo, pescatarian, vegan, or any other form of diet regime to your family's meals. The keto diet is hugely popular right now and, along with the many health benefits it offers, people are finding it makes them feel great. Unfortunately, cutting out major food groups, such as grains, isn't an easy switch for a busy family when kids are so conditioned to having sandwiches, pizza and burgers.

You also need to be careful to make sure your family is getting a balanced diet with all the nutrients that growing bodies need. So, for now we're going to focus on basic rules and making simple tweaks that will improve the health of you and your family.

SO WHAT IS HEALTHY EATING?

Eating healthy is all about making better choices. But, if it was simply that easy, why isn't everyone eating better? Well, that's because we have a complicated relationship with food. Some of us eat when we're feeling depressed as a way to control our lives. Others like the taste of junk food too much to quit it. In fact, our bodies can actually get addicted to fats and sugars. So don't feel bad if the thought of giving up or cutting back on Oreos makes you feel anxious. It's an addiction and you can definitely kick it.

We often eat whatever meals we can make the fastest. Unfortunately, you don't always have the time to cook a homemade meal from scratch every night. This isn't Christmas! You still need to get the kids to finish their homework and take a bath. This is not mentioning the chores around the house that still need done and the quality time with your partner you need to squeeze in before bed. It makes sense that so many people go for the quickest option.

We often live by the golden rule of "I'll start tomorrow." Why else do so many New Year's resolutions to lose weight go unresolved? We push it to the side until we can find time to do it. You're only capable of so much!

Adjust your expectations. If you eat out several times a week because a home cooked meal just isn't in the schedule, then so be it. Instead of forcing yourself to cook every night and pushing yourself to the limit, think of an alternative. If you eat fast food, eat the healthier options. Get a salad or grilled chicken instead of the greasy burger. Order grilled fish instead of battered fish. Eat apple slices instead of fries. If you're trying to eat in more, take turns with your partner cooking meals. If your kids are old enough, have them cook one meal a week. They'll be helping the household while learning a critical life skill.

Take time to enjoy your meal. There's a reason mama bear's porridge was so cold. It's because she spent all of her time preparing everyone else's plate. By the time she sits down to eat her own meal, it's cold and she's rushing through it. When you don't take the time to eat your meal slower, you risk overeating. Worse, you might get heartburn or indigestion. Take the time to enjoy your meal. Savor every bite. Notice the flavor and the textures of the food. What are the colors? Most often we find foods that are yellow or brown look the most appetizing. Now, you're adding mindfulness to your meal.

FOODS TO AVOID

Processed Food

Processed junk food has little to no nutrient benefit and does not play a role in healthy eating. Processed foods cause inflammation in your body. Inflammation is the process your body uses to help heal when you're sick or injured. But if inflammation is a constant state in your body, your risk of heart disease, obesity and diabetes increase.

Most processed foods are full of sugar, preservatives, and trans fats. Not to mention genetically modified foods, which is a whole other topic.

There are trans fats in dairy, beef, veal, lamb and mutton but the trans fats you really need to watch out for are in processed foods. These trans fats are created in the manufacturing process. They make foods crisp and help them last longer but they're a health hazard you really need to avoid.

Trans fats increase your risk of heart disease as they increase "bad" (LDL) cholesterol and reduce your levels of "good" (HDL) cholesterol.

If you must buy processed foods, you can check labels, but know that manufacturers are only required to list total fat and saturated fat. This means labels may not mention trans fats. Instead, watch out for the word "hydrogenated vegetable oils" which are alternative words for trans fats – but it's much easier to just avoid processed foods.

Sugary Items

Too much added sugar in your diet leads to inflammation and insulin resistance (hello Type 2 diabetes), increased "bad" (LDL) cholesterol, obesity, cardiovascular disease, inflammation and increased gut permeability. It also depletes your body of potassium, which is crucial for muscles (including those in your heart and digestive tract) function normally.

Both sugar and high fructose corn syrup, which is often used to add sweetness to food, are inflammatory.

The American Heart Association (AHA) recommends women limit added sugar to 100 calories – about six teaspoons per day or 23 grams. The recommended limit for men is 150 calories, which is about nine teaspoons or 36 grams per day.

OK, I hope you haven't put this book down in disgust after reading that. Who needs more bad news these days? Of course, you need to eliminate sugar from your diet wherever you can. I know it's hard to do this when you have kids. First, they like candy. How many holidays revolve around them eating it? Easter, Halloween, Valentine's Day, and Christmas, to name a few. How can we be expected not to sneak a candy bar from their Halloween bag when they're sleeping? It's called candy tax and we deserve it after walking around the neighborhood for two hours ringing doorbell after doorbell.

Thanks to candy being associated with fun times and used as a reward, most of us have a strong emotional connection to sweet foods from childhood, so I totally understand if cutting sugar from the diet seems impossible.

But it's not all doom and gloom. Here's something that will make you happy: dark chocolate is good for you. Yes, really! A couple of squares of good quality dark chocolate, with at least 70% cocoa, has many health benefits. This food of the gods contains antioxidants and minerals, and has been shown to reduce insulin resistance and inflammation, lower the risk of heart disease, and may even improve brain function. How good is that? Remember dark chocolate still has calories and fats so, to avoid weight gain, don't eat more than one ounce per day.

Another alternative is to substitute sugar with alternatives. Try the following:

- Raw, organic honey. The raw version has not been heat treated. High in minerals and enzymes, honey also has immune-boosting properties.

- Maple syrup (not maple flavoured syrup).
- Coconut Palm Sugar
- Monk Fruit. Very sweet but has no calories and no impact on blood sugar levels.
- Mesquite. High in minerals and soluble fiber. Has a slight nutty flavor.
- Xylitol. This is a natural sweetener found in plant material. It's almost as sweet as sugar but has way fewer calories. It's often found in "sugar free" candies and chewing gum. However, be wary of having too much as it can have a laxative effect!
- Stevia (liquid or powder). Stevia has a slightly unusual flavour but has no calories and does not affect blood sugar levels.

Note: Use honey and maple syrup sparingly as they are high in calories and affect blood sugar levels in a similar way to cane sugar. Unlike cane sugar though, these sugar substitutes are high in minerals.

Pizza

Pizza. Oh, pizza. It tastes so good, yet it can be so bad. I hate to speak ill of pizza when it's had your back so many times. Birthday parties. Office parties. Pretty much any party—pizza is served. Days when you don't feel like cooking or you don't have the time—pizza is there. Even those drunk college nights probably involved pizza. Unfortunately, pizza is greasy, oily, and usually made of processed meat. That's what makes it taste so good. What doesn't feel good is the bloating or inflammation that comes with it. If cutting out pizza is just out of the question, then try making your own pizza with healthier ingredients. You can use special bread for the dough, a low-fat cheese or special sauce, and fresh vegetables. Google recipes for using cauliflower as a pizza base. I've tried it and can report that it actually works very well. You can choose what meat, if any, goes on your pizza. Steer away from cheap processed meats if you can.

Anything White and Fluffy

And I'm not talking fairy floss here. Bread, rice and pasta are favorite comfort foods for many. They're even a strong staple in some diets. Unfortunately, white bread, white rice and white pasta have calories with little nutritional value. Fiber, Vitamin B, and other minerals are also lacking (unless artificially added). Eating these foods will give you short bursts of energy but won't keep you full for long. They also increase the level of blood sugar in your body, contributing to an increased risk of cardiovascular problems.

Instead of the white variety, choose complex carbohydrates such as quinoa or wholemeal that take longer to digest and leave you feeling fuller for longer.

Soda

Not a food, but something we all need to be mindful of is soda drinks. The problem with sugary drinks is that your brain doesn't register the calories that come from them. You're drinking empty calories in addition to your body asking for more calories in the form of food because it didn't account for the ones from the soda.

Here's a scary statistic there are 39 grams or 9 1/3 teaspoons in a 12-ounce can of Coke. Just one can will put you well over the recommended daily limit. So all you will gain from drinking soda is a large helping of added sugar.

And don't think switching to diet soda will be OK. A recent study comparing regular and diet soda concluded that switching to diet soda doesn't lower the risk of diabetes.

Instead of drinking soda every other day, cut back to soda as a weekly treat. Better yet, use seltzer water to replace it. This is where investing in a Soda Stream machine can reap dividends to your wallet as well as your health.

Other Sugary Drinks

Fruit juice is a way to get the nutrient benefits of fruit, but even just one 8oz glass per day can cause sugar spikes. When blood sugar levels "crash" after the spike, it will leave you feeling drained and in need of another sugar hit.

Consumed in the same quantity, the amount of sugar in juice can be even higher than soda. Unsweetened grape juice in the amount equivalent to a can of soda has a whopping 54 grams of sugar. Even orange juice has 32 grams.

Where you can, eat real fruit. You'll consume far less sugar as it will fill you up and you'll get a dose of all-important fiber too.

Other drinks that are best avoided because of the unnecessary amounts of sugar include sports drinks, flavored milk drinks, and bottled iced tea and coffee.

PLANNING MEALS

Think of your home as a business. Not too hard to imagine, right? Well, you're the upper management...,and lower management, as well as a regular employee, too. You pretty much do it all: plan, organize, and manage your household. Like any household, it can be hard keeping up with everything, and sometimes you fall behind. It's okay. It happens to even the best businesses—I mean, households. You just need to refocus and come up with a new plan.

Regarding to the food department, you can plan your meals ahead of time so you aren't standing in the middle of the kitchen, shrugging when your child asks what's for dinner. Plus, having a plan, or backup plan, can help with those days when something unexpected comes up (or those days when you're just too lazy to cook).

A meal planner can help. You can use a chalkboard or whiteboard to keep track of what your plans for dinner will be throughout the week. As a bonus, you can find boards that already have calendars or days of the week to make it easier. If you're like many moms out there, calendars and the illusion that you're organized makes you feel you are, even when you're not. Still, give it a try. You might find it helpful to maintain control of the kitchen.

If you can afford it, you can try a home-delivery option for meal plans. They ship the ingredients in a box with directions. All you need to do is make the food, which these services usually brag is easy to make.

Prep Ahead

This applies on so many levels.

Find out what you're making for the week and figure out what all those ingredients are so you're prepared when you're shopping. Plus, you can avoid so many shopping trips throughout the week to buy items for dinner because you'll already have what you need.

Fix lunchboxes the night before so you aren't scrambling to throw one together five minutes before the bus comes.

Prep meals ahead of time. Make a big bowl of egg salad or chicken salad for an easier lunch. Pre-cut vegetables to cut d0wn on prep time during dinner. You can even chop the vegetables and put them in a sandwich baggie to freeze so they don't go bad as soon.

GLUTEN

This is a hot topic. Anyone who's used the internet in the last decade has probably heard about gluten. It's plastered all over the products at the grocery store: gluten-free this and gluten-free that.

Many people are going gluten free now for the simple reason they feel better avoiding gluten. There's been much talk in the media about this with some medical professionals scoffing at what they see as a health fad. However, if you've tried going gluten-free and found you feel better for it, there is a good reason.

What is Gluten?

So what the heck is gluten? Gluten is a protein found in grains like oats, barley, rye, and wheat, that holds its form like glue.

Gluten is an inflammatory food. Which means it can affect the lining of your gut, making it more permeable. When this happens, larger molecules of food can cross into your bloodstream. This triggers an inflammatory response. You may not notice an immediate , but hours or even days later you may find yourself with symptoms such as:

- Fatigue
- Bloating
- Stomach aches
- Nausea
- Diarrhea
- Brain fog
- Headaches
- Joint or muscle pain

Celiac Disease

Some people are severely intolerant to gluten and have what is called celiac disease. Basically, this is when your immune system mistakes gluten for something dangerous and responds by producing a bunch of antibodies to attack the gluten. Take that, gluten! Unfortunately, it also attacks the lining of your small intestine, and the damage prevents nutrients from being absorbed. Celiac disease is serious and can lead to other serious health issues, including infertility, anemia, osteoporosis and liver disease. Sufferers need to cut gluten completely from their diet permanently.

Cut It Out

Some people find it easier to just avoid gluten. The plus side is that only a small number of people have any major problems with gluten. But even if you aren't diagnosed with celiac disease, it doesn't mean you can't watch your gluten intake.

This is one you can experiment with. Cut out gluten for three weeks and note how you feel. If you've been getting any of the above symptoms and they stop, or you just feel better overall, then you know removing gluten will make you feel better.

The following foods contain gluten:

- Wheat / wheat derivatives
- Rye
- Barley
- Brewer's yeast

Did I lose you? It's all good. Common foods you see with this are:

- Bread
- Pastries
- Biscuits
- Pancakes, crepes, and waffles
- Crackers
- Cereal
- Pasta
- Noodles
- Beer

I bet at least one thing on that list had you crying *nooo!*

Luckily, there are many gluten-free choices at the store now. But keep an eye out for the level of sugar in these foods. As mentioned above, the daily maximum that's recommended for sugar for women is 23 grams.

KEEP RED MEAT TO A MINIMUM

Red meat is another inflammatory food. There are many studies showing red meat (lamb, beef and pork) consumption is associated with risk of diseases.

For example, a 2017 study carried out by the National Cancer Institute in Maryland, US, and published in the British Medical Journal, concluded that meat consumption increases the risk of cancer, type 2 diabetes, stroke, infections, and diseases of the kidneys, heart, respiratory tract, and liver. The same study also showed reduced risks when white meat (poultry and fish), particularly unprocessed white meat, was eaten instead.

BE WARY OF DAIRY

Cow's milk is great for baby cows—who have four stomachs to do the digesting. Unfortunately, it isn't so easy for humans to digest. Humans are the only mammals who drink another mammal's milk—and way beyond the baby stage when it's required.

On top of that, cows may be fed genetically modified feed, antibiotics and hormones to increase milk production. If you drink milk or eat dairy products, you will consume these chemicals.

Some people react to milk as they do not have the lactase enzyme necessary to breakdown the lactose sugar it contains. Other people react to the milk proteins.

Sometimes reactions to milk are not obvious. If you're wondering if your body is digesting milk properly, try eliminating it for at least three weeks and see how you feel. If it turns out to be an issue, there are many other options. Try other milks, such as rice milk or nut milks.

AVOID UNWANTED CHEMICALS

Much of the food you buy from the supermarket has chemicals that are best avoided. Commercial farming methods rely on pesticides in order to grow fruit and vegetables, while processed and packaged foods have all kinds of chemicals to preserve, add color, or enhance flavor.

While always eating fresh food means you don't have to check labels, there are probably several items you buy pre-prepared.

The following list is pretty long but if you're serious about wanting the best for your family's health it's worth checking that you are avoiding or at least minimizing these main toxic chemicals:

1. Monosodium Glutamate (MSG/e621)
2. A flavor enhancer used in Chinese food, potato chips, cookies, seasonings, lunch meats and frozen dinners. This evil little chemical affects the neurological pathways of the brain and switches off the "I'm full" function, which can cause weight gain. Eating MSG too often may result in fatigue, headaches, depression, disorientation, and obesity. Note: small amounts may not be declared on labels.
3. Food Dyes (e133 / e124 / e110/ e102)
4. You've probably heard of, or worse still experienced, children going hyper after red cordial. There are a number of artificial colors that can contribute to behavioral problems like hyperactivity, ADD, and ADHD. Unfortunately, these food dyes crop up in many products such as breakfast cereals, soft drinks, ice cream, sauces, peanut butter and candy. Particular culprits to watch out for are Red #40, Yellow #5 (Tartrazine), Yellow #6 (Sunset Yellow), Blue #2 and sodium benzoate.
5. Sulphur Dioxide (e220)
6. This is a toxic additive used as a preservative in wine, beer, soft drinks, vinegar, dried fruit, juices, cordials, and potato products. It may cause reactions such as asthma, bronchial problems, flushing tingling sensations, hypotension, or anaphylactic shock.
7. Aspartame (e951).
8. Aspartame is a neurotoxin (affects nervous system) and a carcinogen (causes cancer). Consumption can lead to diabetes, headaches, nausea, depression, anxiety, dizziness, chronic fatigue, mental confusion, Alzheimer's Disease, Parkinson's Disease, fibromyalgia, lymphoma, multiple sclerosis, depression, and seizures. Watch out for aspartame in "diet" or "sugar free" products, including tabletop sweeteners, diet coke, coke zero, cereal, desserts, sugar free gum, drink mixes, iced tea, toothpaste, chewable vitamins, and cough syrup.
9. Sodium Sulphite (e221)

10. A preservative used in wine and dried fruit like raisins or sultanas. Around 1% of the population is sensitive to sulphites, which can cause headaches, asthma, rashes and breathing problems.
11. BHA and BHT (e320 / 321)
12. These are common preservatives used in candy, jello, cereal, lard, shortening, potato chips, and gum. They can affect the neurological system of the brain and alter behavior. Both BHA and BHT are oxidants, which form cancer-causing reactive compounds in your body.
13. Aluminum Additives
14. Food that is stored in aluminum foil or cooked in aluminum baking foil may contain traces of aluminum. Aluminum can have neurological effects on behavioral, motor, and learning functions. It is also associated with Alzheimer's disease and other neurodegenerative conditions.
15. Sodium Nitrate (e250)
16. This chemical is used in a range of processed meats, including ham, bacon, luncheon meat, cured meats, and corned beef. It can also be found in smoked fish. It's a cancer-causing chemical that can cause problems with many internal organs, in particular the liver and pancreas in particular.
17. Potassium Bromate (e924)
18. This chemical is used to increase volume in breads and is known to cause cancer in animals.
19. Propyl Paraben (e216)
20. A preservative found in baked foods and dyes. It's a hormone disrupter that's also linked to accelerated cancer growth.

OK, so we've been through a lot of things to avoid. If you're still with me, congratulations on making it to the best part of this chapter. The following is a guide for making sure your diet is as healthy as possible without being too draconian.

EAT MORE RAW FRUITS AND VEGETABLES

Full of nutrients that will benefit your body, tasty and little preparation required. What's not to love? Raw food has more nutrients, as the vitamins and minerals have not been destroyed by cooking.

Alternatives to eating vegetables raw include light steaming and slow cooking to preserve as many nutrients as possible.

But let's be practical here. Your kid is going to be more than a little dismayed when he opens his lunchbox to find raw celery and carrot sticks. You may need to stick to sandwiches in the lunchbox and find other ways to get the vegetables into him.

Try disguising them by blending them together to create interesting smoothie drinks. You can add raw cacao and honey to make it taste like a chocolate smoothie with no hint of the spinach lurking inside.

"What's with the pond slime?" was the most frequent question I used to get when I started making green smoothies many years ago. Now the funny looks have stopped and you can buy green juices and smoothies over the counter at kiosks and cafes.

The beauty of green juices and smoothies is they're a great tasting way to get a good daily serving of raw fruits and vegetables. In particular, the dark leafy ones that can be , especially to kids.

I won't go into a whole set of menus here as there are loads of great books, e-books and free recipes all over the internet on how to make smoothies. But if you're interested, here's one of my favorites as it's so simple and quick. Throw the following ingredients into a high-speed blender:

- Coconut water
- Handful of raw baby spinach leaves
- 1 medium carrot
- 1 small apple
- 1/2 frozen banana
- Teaspoon of organic cacao powder

Blend on high for around 20 seconds. That's it basically. Sometimes

I add some frozen organic blueberries for a change, but I keep this to just a few so it doesn't become too sweet.

EATING ORGANIC

Minimizing pesticides and genetically modified foods is the way to go for your health. But eating exclusively organic can be expensive. Especially if you live in a city and buy from a local organic shop.

If cost or availability are issues, you can start by replacing some items on the "dirty dozen" list, which are the fruits and vegetables that have the most traces of pesticides.

The Environmental Working Group (EWG) regularly updates its "Dirty Dozen". list. For 2022 the fruit and vegetables you should buy organic, where possible are:

1. Strawberries
2. Spinach
3. Kale
4. Nectarines
5. Apples
6. Grapes
7. Bell and hot peppers
8. Cherries
9. Peaches
10. Pears
11. Celery
12. Tomatoes

The EWG also produces a "Clean 15". List, which are the fruits and vegetables that are less likely to be contaminated. So you can feel better about buying these non-organic as there is less potential for them to be contaminated.

The Clean 15 for 2022 are:

1. Avocados
2. Sweet Corn

3. Pineapple
4. Onions
5. Papaya
6. Sweet Peas (frozen)
7. Asparagus
8. Honeydew Melon
9. Kiwi
10. Cabbage
11. Mushrooms
12. Cantaloupe
13. Mangoes
14. Watermelon
15. Sweet Potatoes

HINTS FROM THE MEDITERRANEAN DIET

If you want direction on what sort of food you can incorporate into your family's diet, you can't go past the Mediterranean diet. It's relatively easy to follow, allows for delicious recipes and has proven health benefits. A recent study showed the Mediterranean diet is good for brain health, which is so important, particularly as we get older.

In summary, to follow the Mediterranean diet:

- Eat mainly plant-based foods including fruit, vegetables, whole grains, legumes and nuts.
- Eat fish and chicken at least twice/week
- Limit red meat to 2–3 times/month
- Use healthy fats such as olive oil (rather than butter)
- Use herbs and spices for flavor (instead of salt)
- Enjoy red wine in moderation (if you feel like it).

Note: Where you can, eat wild caught fish rather than farmed fish, which may have been given genetically modified feed. And, of course, free range chicken is a far kinder option.

Benefits of the Mediterranean diet:

- Help prevent cardiovascular disease
- Improve brain health
- Reduce risk of Alzheimer's Disease
- Prevent/manage diabetes
- Improve mood
- Protect against cancer

As well as providing a framework for foods to eat, the Mediterranean way of eating involves everyone in the family sitting down to eat together. Making mealtimes a time to connect in this way fulfils social needs and provides an opportunity for family bonding.

Note: avoid regularly eating large fish such as tuna, orange roughy, shark, swordfish and king mackerel, as these can contain mercury. Pregnant or nursing women should avoid these altogether.

PINPOINT FOODS YOUR BODY DOESN'T LIKE

Allergies and sensitivities to different foods are common. While there are differences between allergies and sensitivities, both have a negative effect on your health. If you suspect you have an allergy or sensitivity, consult a health practitioner. Keep a food diary for three weeks, noting the foods you eat and the symptoms you have. Sensitivities are often not immediate. In fact it can take up to three days for some reactions to manifest, so it may take some experimentation to find out what foods are causing issues.

YOUR HEALTH IS IN YOUR HANDS

A stitch in time saves … your health and wellbeing.

We all have genetic predispositions to various ailments and diseases. The good news is we don't have to be at the mercy of our genes. We can switch off "bad" genes and switch on the "good" ones when we have a healthy diet and environment.

A paper published in 2017 in the American Journal of Medical Genetics describes how the activation or silencing of genes by environmental factors such as diet, gut microbiota, and infections plays a significant role in disease manifestation.

Which means you don't have to manifest the same ailments your parents and grandparents had. Taking care to eat a healthy diet is one of the major important steps to help avoid developing conditions that run in families and protect your health and wellbeing.

CHAPTER TAKEAWAYS

- Too much sugar makes you feel sluggish, is bad for your health, and makes you gain weight.
- Pizza. While it tastes good and is convenient, it's greasy and often made with fattening or unhealthy ingredients. Try making a healthier pizza if you don't want to give it up.
- Prepping dinner ahead of time can be a stress reliever, particularly if you've had a busy day and don't want fast food *again*. Try planning meals so you can buy your groceries all at once. Plan it on a board in the kitchen, where you don't need to spend time figuring out what to make.
- Gluten is a common cause of feeling tired and sluggish. Try cutting it out for three weeks and see how you feel.
- Keep red meat to a minimum.
- Be wary of dairy.
- Avoid unwanted chemicals.
- Eat more raw fruits and vegetables—preferably organic.
- Check out the Mediterranean Diet, which has proven health benefits.
- Pinpoint foods your body doesn't like.

CHAPTER 7
MOVE THAT BODY MAMA

"When it comes to health and well-being, regular exercise is about as close to a magic potion as you can get." Thich Nhat Hanh

Exercise. For some, it's a cursed word. After spending the day working, cleaning, cooking, and taking care of your family, you're supposed to exercise? How's that possible when you can barely keep your eyes open? Motherhood is exhausting, so it makes sense that many women lose their exercise routine when they have kids. Where's the time?

Why should you exercise?

- Exercise releases endorphins, the happy hormone. Being active will make you happy.
- You'll build your confidence. After having kids, you might not feel as sexy as before. Your body changes; it's only natural. Even if you don't keep the baby weight, there may still be scars to remind you of your child's birth. , C-section scars, even a higher shoe size—these are all physical reminders of your pregnancy that can sometimes leave a hit to your self-esteem.

- Movement is a form of meditation. Let your mind clear and the stress melt away.
- You'll build your immune system. This is so important at this time in the world where viruses are wreaking havoc.
- Exercise will make you energized. I know it's ironic, considering you should feel tired from exercise, but in the long run, you won't feel so exhausted in your daily life and you'll fall asleep easier at night. In other words, you'll be tired when you need to be and energetic when it counts.
- You'll lose weight and gain muscle. It's no secret that women are conscious of their weight. You're either too thin or too fat. Sometimes it feels like women can never just look good the way they are. At least, that's what society tries to tell us. Why else is the "dad bod" trending but the "mom bod" is nonexistent? The truth is, if you want to lose weight, it should be because you want to feel healthier and not to live up to some unrealistic standard. Remember, even Aphrodite —goddess of love—had curves.
- If nothing else, you get to wear yoga pants.

SET GOALS

Starting a new exercise regimen can be daunting. Where do you start? Well, you want to lose 20 pounds, but how do you get there? You've been exercising for month and have barely made progress. Don't feel discouraged. You're looking at this from the wrong perspective.

Instead of checking every day to see if that 2o pounds has disappeared, set a smaller, more achievable goal for yourself. Make your goals realistic and attainable.

Start off with a simple goal, like drinking eight glasses of water a day. If you need help keeping track of your water intake, you can buy a plastic tumbler with a water tracker to help. These tumblers have times labeled on the side to ensure you're drinking enough, so all you need to do is fill it up and drink it on time.

Your next goal could be to cut out soda from your diet. If you're an avid soda drinker, limit it to one soda a day until you can comfortably replace it with water or tea. Maybe soda isn't your weakness. Does a bowl of ice cream before bed or a donut with breakfast sound more like you? Try reducing your sugar intake wherever possible.

After that, make it a goal to walk ten minutes around your neighborhood after dinner. You can do this by yourself, with a friend, or with the family, as long as you're taking a short walk every day.

Slowly make your goals harder to attain. It shouldn't be so difficult that you're set up for failure, but you want the goal to be a challenge, something you feel proud of achieving. By starting small and working your way up, you're making it possible to achieve your goals. Think of it like building muscle. You don't start by lifting the heavy weights; you try the five-pound weights, then the ten-pound ones, and slowly increase until you reach the heavy weights.

MEASURE PROGRESS

Keep a journal that measures your progress. You can write down your goals and work toward them. Then you can look back at the progress you've made, which helps when you're struggling with a challenging goal. Alternatively, you can make a vision board of your goals. Hang it in sight to keep you motivated.

You should measure your progress based on how you feel and not by the number on the scale. Has adding exercise to your life made you feel healthier? Eating more fruits and vegetables will make you feel stronger and build your immunity. All those sugars you would previously eat are now replaced by something more nutritious, which makes you feel less exhausted than usual. This is the progress you should measure. Keeping track of your weight is good, but it shouldn't be the only focus.

USE SOCIAL MEDIA

YouTube Videos

Going to the gym isn't always the answer to staying fit. Maybe the idea of working out in front of people who are already in shape is a turnoff or you can't afford the cost of a gym. Memberships are expensive, and many families live paycheck to paycheck. YouTube videos are a great way to have a guided workout in the comfort of your own home (and without witnesses to your attempt at physical fitness).

You can find videos for every level and type of fitness. You can even make it something you do with the kids. If your toddler won't give you time during the day to work out, find a "mommy and me" video. Then you can be active while entertaining your child and ensuring they stay active, too.

Social Media Groups

Join a group on social media. Whether it's a Facebook group or a forum from your favorite parenting website, you can join in with others to stay fit. You can motivate others to keep up with their fitness, and they can do the same for you. Plus, if you announce a goal, such as losing ten pounds this month, you'll be more likely to keep up with your goal to avoid the shame of not meeting it. Another benefit of joining a group is that other moms can give you advice or tell you what worked for them.

Work Out With Other Moms

It helps to have others around you who are also trying to be healthy. Do you have a mom friend who wants to get into shape, also? Maybe you guys can work out together. While the kids are at school, you can jog to the local coffee shop and then talk while you sip on a cup of Joe. Keep up with each other's progress and motivate each other to accomplish your goals.

Use Your Phone

There are plenty of apps available to help you track your weight loss and fitness goals. Try an app that acts as a personal trainer and coaches you through your sessions. Is jogging your preference? There are apps that map routes and track your speed and distance when you run.

HOW TO INCLUDE EXERCISE IN YOUR BUSY SCHEDULE

Make it a Family Affair

Do something active as a family. It can be an event like a family outing or something simple, like taking a walk together. The point is, you're getting a workout in while spending time with your family. Plus, you're helping to keep them active, as well. Let's face it—that's not as easy as it used to be now that there's electronics to keep them rooted to the couch.

Here are few ideas to help you get active together:

- Bowling
- Mini-golf
- Hiking
- Playing a sport like soccer, softball, basketball, or football
- Dancing—even if it's in the living room
- Walking around the neighborhood
- Biking

Get another family involved. If you have friends with kids, set up a game of kickball or capture the flag. There are plenty of games you can play. Just think back to the games you played in school when you were a child, like Four Square, Red Rover, or Red Light Green Light. Playing with another family also gives yours a chance to bond by working as a team.

Squeeze It in Where You Can

Sometimes, the only way you can exercise is if you squeeze it in where you can. If you take the bus as transportation, get off at a stop earlier to extend your walk. Take your lunch break outside and take a stroll around the block. While you're watching television, try doing a few squats or sit-. If you have the option, ride your bike to get around town. Walk to the grocery store instead of driving there. When you take out the garbage, take a walk around the block. The kids can come with you and hopefully tire themselves out for an easier bedtime. You can also turn their playtime into dance time. That can wear them out, too.

Exercise doesn't always need to be a grueling workout session at the gym. Even these small ways of fitting it into your schedule can make a difference and also get you into the habit of being active. You just need to take the opportunity when you see it.

CHAPTER TAKEAWAYS

- Exercise:
- It releases endorphins and makes you happy.
- It builds confidence and raises your self-esteem.
- It's a form of meditation. Clear your mind and reduce your stress: what a bonus!
- It builds immunity: Try to get you now, pesky germs!
- It makes you feel energized and fall asleep easier.
- It helps you lose weight and feel healthier.
- You get to wear yoga pants!
- Start small and work your way up. It's less daunting that way and you're more likely to be successful.
- Start drinking more water. Move up to cutting out sugar. Then add in some short walks.
- Make your goals and expectations realistic.
- Keep a journal and write down your goals and accomplishments.
- Make a vision board of your goals and keep it in plain sight to motivate you.
- Remember, it's about how you feel, not the number on the scale. Losing weight is good, but feeling healthy is better.
- Watch YouTube exercise videos from the comfort of your living room. You'll have free guided workouts. Watch a

mommy and me workout video if you can't get away from the kids. Keeps them healthy, too.

- Join a group online. Talk to other moms with the same goals as you. Help each other stay motivated and reach each other's goals.
- Have a workout buddy. It can be another mom friend with similar fitness goals. Go hiking together, join a sports team, or whatever activity you two are interested in.
- Use your phone. Download apps to help you track your progress and keep you on the right track.
- Turn it into a family affair. Have an outing where you do an activity. Play a sport together. Go hiking or biking. Join another family you're friends with and have teams. This will also let your family bond and work together.
- Squeeze it in where you can. If you don't have time, slip in exercise whenever you have the opportunity. Walk to the store, do squats when you're watching television, get off the bus at a stop early. Walk around the block when you take the trash out.

CHAPTER 8
ALWAYS REMEMBER: YOU ARE IMPERFECTLY PERFECT

"Wanting to be someone else is a waste of the person you are." Marilyn Monroe

We all strive to be the perfect mother. Appearing like we have everything together. Caring and kind, but with a firm hand when we need one. But so often we feel like we fall short. And when we don't meet our own expectations, it can make us feel like a failure.

I love that quote from Marilyn as she sums it up perfectly. You're perfect as you are, doing your best, and that is what matters.

LOVE YOUR BODY

Body image is a tough subject for any woman, mom or not. Whatever age you are, there's always the pressure to look beautiful and compare yourself to other women. When you're young, you wear makeup, style your hair, and wait for your boobs to come in. You get older; you have a baby, and suddenly you're worried about losing that baby weight and getting your old figure back. As if you haven't suffered enough from the demanding beauty standards, your senior years are spent trying to color your gray hair and get rid of your wrinkles. Do we ever catch a break?

Why is it so easy for us to look at another woman and tell her how beautiful she is, regardless of what standards she believes she fails to meet? We can look her in the eyes and say, "You're beautiful the way you are." Yet, when we look at ourselves in the mirror, we can only see the flaws.

You need to love yourself the way you tell other women to. Love yourself the way you deserve to be loved. So what if you have broad shoulders or stubby legs? Does having a belly make you any less of a woman? Forget the eczema that keeps resurfacing on your skin or that mole that stands out on the side of your face.

Do you ever say you wish you were as fat as you thought you were in high school? In other words, you thought you were so unattractive back then, but now you realize how wrong you were and would give anything to be "the fat you thought you were." Imagine another twenty years and the imperfections you think you have now. You'll be thinking, "Man, I wish I looked like that still."

Embrace your imperfections. Quit telling yourself you're not delicate enough, thin enough, tall enough, short enough, or beautiful enough. Your body is unique. It's perfect for you. Besides, how boring would it be if we all had the same "beautiful" mold? It's our differences that make us special. Embrace those differences. Love your body for what it is. Trust me; you'll feel a lot happier and much more confident when you do. If we're going to be scrutinized for our body, no matter what we do, we might as well enjoy what we've been given.

THREE RULES TO LIVE BY

Never Compare Yourself to Others

People tend to compare themselves to others around them. Watch out for that little voice in your head that is all too quick to point out hoe you're failing. If any of the below examples resonate, you need a stern word with yourself:

I've been looking for a house for months and have struggled to find anything decent while this person is buying that quaint cottage by the lake. I've been working so hard at some crappy, low-paying job for years while this person is being promoted. I've been watching my diet for months and haven't made progress while this person who eats whatever they want without gaining weight.

It's not fair.

That seems to be the motto when you compare yourself to others. "It's not fair." Why isn't it? You don't know what struggles and sacrifices they've had to make to get to where they are. That house they bought, the cute cottage they've been sharing pictures of for the last week? They spent the last five years rebuilding their credit and saving up for a down payment. That promotion they got? They spent hours of overtime and listening to someone belittle their work to get that promotion. That person who can eat whatever they want without gaining weight? Well, maybe they just lucked out with a high metabolism.

My point is that the grass may always *seem* greener on the other side, but you don't know how much that person has watered and cared for that grass.

Social media has a lot to answer for too when it comes to our self-esteem. I know, it might seem like that mom on Facebook is perfect. Their house is always spotless, they take their family on vacations, and they are always smiling. And how do they *always* have time to cook a homemade meal with every member of the food group? You must remember: You're only seeing a picture they posted on social media. They might have spent hours cleaning their house before taking that picture. Perhaps that homemade meal was actually store bought and reheated. You're only seeing the part of their life they want you to see. The rest is covered with a silly Snapchat filter.

It's like looking through the window into a beautiful house. From the outside, the white picket fence and rose bushes make the exterior look incredible. If you look hard enough, you'll see the cracks in the foundation. Peek into the window and see that the floor needs replaced and the walls need to be painted.

Don't waste your time feeling sorry for yourself because you aren't at that point in your life that someone else is at. Instead, celebrate with them and feel happy that they have achieved what they have.

Wouldn't you want the same treatment? Plus, it will feel better for the both of you.

Forgive Yourself

Stephanie Lahart beautifully said, "You owe it to yourself to LIVE! Live your life without the regrets, without the resentments, without the unforgiveness, without the blame game, without the self-pity, without any and everything that keeps you from experiencing true joy within! You are too important to waste your life away! Learn to appreciate and value your life, but most importantly, learn to appreciate and value yourself! You count too, no matter what you've done!"

We've all made decisions that weren't our most shining moments to display. We've all made choices we might regret later down the line. It's okay. You're only human. The important thing is to learn from your mistakes. Even things that ended badly offer an outlook on life you can learn from.

Forgive yourself. Love yourself. Allow yourself to embrace your mistakes and look back with a newfound wisdom. You give other people a second chance, so why not give yourself one, too?

Stop Negative Self-Talk

We are so much harder on ourselves than we are on others. So, you spent the day enthralled in a book and ran out of time to make dinner? Don't spend the rest of the night shaming yourself for being a "bad mom." Order takeout and move on. You forgot to set the alarm and now the kids are late for school? Instead of beating yourself up for making a mistake, think of the positives: You got some extra sleep. Every cloud has a silver lining.

TIPS TO CULTIVATE A POSITIVE ATTITUDE

Gratitude

It's important to be grateful for what you have. So often, we focus our energy on what we don't have and what we want. Instead, turn that energy around. Think about all you have and why you are grateful to have it.

Develop a Proper Morning Routine

How you begin your morning can set your mood for the entire day. Don't wake up irritated and annoyed. It will set the tone for the rest of the day. You want to start your day with positivity. Eat breakfast, take a shower, drink some coffee—whatever it takes to make your day start off right. If necessary, set your alarm 15 minutes early and spend a few minutes breathing deeply, meditating, stretching or simply planning your day so you feel less frazzled.

Close Your Lips, Chatty Cathy

Avoid gossip and speaking negatively about people. It only reflects your character, which isn't living up to the best version of yourself that you want to be. You don't want to be that person who spreads negativity at the expense of others. Learn to give compliments to others and spread love, not rumors.

Lighten Up

Laughter is the best medicine. It lifts your mood and lets you feel positive and light. When you feel good, you're able to hold on to that positivity you so desperately want.

Listen to Music

Music has always been a great source for soothing your wounds and calming your mind. When you're feeling sad, you listen to somber music. When you're happy, you want to sing along to the bounciest pop song you know. Music can lift your mood and help you process your emotions. Music is there for the moments of heartbreak, joy, anger, excitement, and every other emotion you feel.

Focus on Long-Term Goals Over Short-Term Occurrences

In times of conflict, take a minute to think if it is worth reacting and getting defensive, especially with your family. It could be a bad day for your kids or husband. In these times, before you hit them back with a scathing response, think about whether it is worth ruining your mood over a small momentary conflict. Anger will not help you solve the problem at all. Instead, learn to focus on the bigger picture and analyze if such a response is even worth it. Exercise more empathy and less anger.

CHAPTER TAKEAWAYS

- Never compare yourself to others. It will only make you feel bad about yourself. Everyone lives their life at a different pace, and thinking the grass is greener on their side doesn't make your grass any less vibrant. Besides, you don't know the care they put into making their grass green.
- Forgive yourself. We allow other's forgiveness easier than we do for ourselves. Forgive yourself and the mistakes you make. You're only human.
- Stop the negative self-talk. Think positive and you will see positive things happen around you. However, thinking negatively about everything will only result in being surrounded by negativity.
- Show gratitude for what you have. You might not have a fancy new car, but your beat-up van gets you where you need to go. Appreciate what you have and who you are.
- Start the day off right. If you start on a happy note, you'll have a happier day.

- Don't gossip and talk about others. Focus on your own life and only spread positivity when you speak of others.
- Lighten up and laugh a little. It will make you feel so much better.
- Listening to music can make you feel happier. If you need to turn up the heavy metal and scream, then do it (taking care not to wake the sleeping baby or traumatize the toddler of course!).
- Instead of focusing on negative things, redirect that focus to a more positive thinking.

CHAPTER 9
SOCIAL CONNECTION IS A BASIC HUMAN NEED

"We seek fulfillment in our lives through heart connection with others. This is our soul's essence of joy, which spontaneously pulses through us, longing to share itself with another." John Friend

Humans are social beings by nature. We're pack animals, and without our pack, we're lost. Just a lonely little wolf scraping by to survive.

We need a community to thrive. It gives us purpose and makes us less isolated. We're a part of something larger than ourselves. When we're denied these connections, we lose our sense of belonging and can easily become depressed. Why else do people use solitary confinement as punishment?

That's why building connections is vital to our existence. Being alienated from the rest of the world can make us feel like happiness is slowly being sucked out of us. Sure, there are times when we wish we could hide from our kids to get a moment of time to ourselves, but sometimes we need that connection to someone else.

WAYS TO CONNECT

Having a family can make it hard to keep in touch with your friends. Life happens. People move, they start a life elsewhere, and they stay busy with all the demands of day-to-day living. Before you know it, months or even years have gone by without talking. Don't take it personally. You're probably doing the same thing to them. It's hard to fit a social life into your busy schedule. So, how *can* you stay social when you stay busy?

Stay in Touch

It can be awkward to get in touch with someone you haven't spoken to in a while. They might refrain from sending you a message or an email because they're feeling the same way. Push past it. Don't feel anxious about sending a quick: "Hey, how are you doing?" Sending even a brief message can really make someone's day because that means you're thinking of them. We all want to know that people care about us and think about us from time to time. It makes us feel special. Let me give you an example.

Amelia was nearing her 30th birthday. Her husband and two children wanted to make the day special, but no matter what they did, Amelia couldn't shake the feeling of depression. It wasn't her age that was bothering her, like her husband thought. He figured she was upset that she was entering a new decade, but the truth was that she was feeling isolated. She'd always wanted to have a big party for her 30th with her friends and family there to celebrate and even wanted it to be "Friends" themed (the one where they turn 30).

The problem was that they moved to another state and didn't live near her friends and family. Usually, she would keep up with everyone on Facebook, commenting on pictures of their kids and fun outings. But with her birthday approaching and no way of seeing the people she was close to, she became withdrawn. Suddenly, those pictures were hard to look at. It felt like everyone was moving on in the world while she was standing still. Everyone was continuing with their lives, making new friendships, and going on adventures without her.

It was too painful to know everyone had moved on. It was like they didn't even care. Sure, people would comment when she posted and would leave hearts on pictures of her family, but they wouldn't really talk to her. Not like they used to. If they weren't going to take the time to talk to her, why should she bother? So, she deleted her Facebook profile without a word to anyone.

She hadn't deleted the Messenger app because she still used that to talk to her husband and a few family members. A few weeks after deleting Facebook, she got a message from her friend, Bethany, asking if she was doing okay. She noticed Amelia hadn't been posting for a while and wanted to check in on her.

That message meant everything to Amelia because it felt so good to know that her friends thought of her, despite their lack of conversation. Bethany noticed Amelia's absence.

Sometimes, sending a quick message can really make a difference.

Be the Bigger Person

Let people know you need them. Don't be afraid to be vulnerable around those you love. If you have a disagreement, be the bigger person and apologize. I'm not saying to let someone walk all over you, but don't let your pride cloud your reasoning. Ask yourself: Is it worth potentially losing a friendship?

Communicate With the People You Love

Ask them about their day and how they've been doing. Talk to them about their life. Sometimes, your friends need someone to listen to them. I know, with everything going on, you need to vent to someone outside of your family. It's the same for your friends. They need to vent, too, and if you're the one who's always doing the talking, they might not want to spend as much time with you.

MEETING NEW PEOPLE

I know the idea of meeting new people sounds intimidating. It's uncomfortable and slightly terrifying. We all have this desire to be accepted by people, and making new friends is a vulnerable experience. Can you trust them? Will they like you for you? What if they think your unorthodox sense of humor is weird? It's like high school all over again.

Find Common Ground

One of the best ways to make new friends is to find common ground. What are your interests? Take a class or join a club relating to it. Join a local mom group and bond with other moms feeling just as isolated as you. Maybe their kids are the same age and they can have a play date while you guys talk over coffee (or wine). At least you have a conversation starter. You can talk about whatever interest you two share that led to your meeting.

Keep an Open Mind and Be Approachable

Approaching someone is nerve-wrecking! You might feel a connection with someone and think, *wow, we could be good friends*, but never take it further because your anxiety is pushing you away. Don't let it. Just walk up to them and ask them to hang out. What's the worst that can happen? They'll say no? Hey, at least you tried, even if you get rejected. If at first you don't succeed, try, try again (with someone else).

In contrast, you want to be approachable, too. Don't hold onto your frown; let it go and allow others to feel comfortable enough to approach you. Body language speaks volumes. If you wear a smile instead of a scowl, they might ask you to hang out.

CONNECT WITH YOUR PARTNER

Always make time to connect with your partner. Your friends are , but your partner is the one you share your life with. They're the one you come home to and sleep next to. You laugh and cry together and share the most intimate moments of your life together. Never stop letting them know how much you appreciate them. Not just for what they do, but for their existence. You're happy that they're around.

Talk to them about their day. Never stop trying to know them. Learn as much about them as you can. Even ten years later, you'll still learn things about your partner that you never knew. Some of it might be good and some of it bad. That's the way it goes. You should know by now that they'll have qualities you don't like, but you're willing to look past them because you love them.

Spend time together. Start a new hobby together or take a class. It doesn't matter what you do, as long as it's something you do together. It doesn't even need to be something new. That suggestion was merely to add a little excitement to your life. As you know, life can get a little mundane (as can your relationship). Keep things interesting with new activities. That includes the more intimate ones, as well.

CHAPTER TAKEAWAYS

- Stay in touch! Even if you haven't talked to your best friend in a year, get in touch with them. It might feel awkward, but it's worth it.
- Be the bigger person. If you have an argument, apologize. Be the bigger person. Step up to the plate. However, don't let people walk all over you. Admit when you're wrong.
- Communicate with the people you love. A little communication goes a long way. Make sure you keep the lines of communication open with the people you love. If they're hurting you, let them know. If you think they're fantastic, tell them.
- Find something you have in common when meeting new people. Join a club of your favorite hobby so you know you have something in common.
- Keep an open mind. Be open to meeting new people. Be someone they feel comfortable approaching.
- Always communicate with your partner. Take time to talk with them and get to know them all over again.

CHAPTER 10

SIMPLIFY AND SMELL THE ROSES

"Enjoy the little things for one day. You may look back and realize they were the big things." Robert Brault.

The problem with being busy is we get so absorbed in dealing with life that we forget to take a moment to appreciate it. It might sound cheesy to say "Sit back and smell the roses," but it's true. If you just take a moment to enjoy what's around you, it can change your life in ways that you'd never imagine.

It really is the little things that make life. Take Renee and her story of how enjoying the small things made her family's vacation an unforgettable one.

Renee had just graduated from college and took a small vacation with her family to celebrate. Four years of keeping up with school, work, children, and home life left her entire family feeling burnt out. After all, this decision to go back to school affected everyone. She wanted to show her family how much she appreciated their support by giving them all a break for a few days.

They decided to take a trip to an underground gorge in the next state over. They would stay two nights at a hotel and visit the gorge on their second day. The drive was only a few hours away, so luckily she avoided the cries of "Are we there yet?" from the kids. Unfortunately, it rained the entire way there and continued to rain throughout the trip.

They got to the hotel and found out there was no internet and the cable was basic. There were no pools or amenities, and the location was in the middle of nowhere. I mean, the closest McDonald's was almost an hour away! Needless to say, some people might think this would make for a dull trip. But not Renee and her family.

Luckily, there was a dollar store close by. They took a trip into town—which was little more than a few streets and a school—and drove around, admiring everything they saw. "Look at that house! That fence is so cute!" "Do you think that fudge shop will be open tomorrow before we leave?" They pointed out the things they liked about the charming houses, imagining what their future dream home would look like.

After they traveled through the whole town, they stopped off at the dollar store. They let each kid pick out a toy and grabbed a knock-off version of Jenga to play at the hotel. There was only one food place in town that was open, and it was a Dairy Queen. Sure, it wasn't some special place and they have a Dairy Queen at home, but that wouldn't stop them from making the most of this trip. They let the kids order whatever they wanted, milkshakes and all. It made the occasion fun and special. They took their food back to the hotel and spent the next few hours munching on Dairy Queen and snacks from the vending machines while playing knock-off Jenga on the uneven table. And they had fun. Without the internet. Without a bustling city life or crazy activities.

The biggest lesson you can learn from self-care is that the smallest things have the biggest impact on your life. Something as small as taking the time to talk to a friend or go for a run can drastically alter your life, and you need to understand that it's the small things in life that truly make life worth living. As a mother, you may expect huge things to happen or wait for milestones, like the day your kid goes to school for the first time, to feel like the experience is truly worth it. But it's really the small things that make us feel the best.

Try to think of the most important moments in your life and you'll find that you always go back to the slightest gestures, the minor details, and the most underrated emotions.

Spending time with your kids and just getting to know them is a great way to smell the roses. You might feel you're only a good mom when you take your kids to a fair or an amusement park, but sometimes just talking with them is all it takes to appreciate them. Find out who they are. You might be amazed at how much you don't know about a person, despite changing their diapers and caring for every aspect of their life.

You can also appreciate the world by getting away from everyone, too. Take a moment for yourself to breathe in the fresh air and just look up at the sky. The way the colors blend can leave you in awe.

CHAPTER TAKEAWAYS

- Enjoy the little things. These are what make the biggest impact on your life.
- Take time to get to know your children. Enjoy just sitting with them and coloring or talking.
- Enjoy the big milestones, but appreciate the small ones, too. Sometimes we get so caught up in "the first day of school" or "the first school dance" that we don't notice the small things.
- Appreciate the world in silence and isolation. Take a moment by yourself to appreciate the colors blended in the sky at sunset, or the crisp, fresh air by the water.

AFTERWORD

To wrap up, let me tell you the story of a mother with whom I was friends. She constantly seemed like she had it all together. Whenever I met her, it would be all smiles, and she would talk about how perfect her life was. I thought nothing was wrong with her life. Then, one day, she called me over to her house, and I found her having a panic attack because she couldn't sew her daughter's Halloween costume.

To see her like that made me realize how close we all are to breaking down. It takes something as small as not being able to thread the needle on the machine to make you suddenly blow up. Once I calmed her down, she explained to me how she had been repressing all her negative emotions because she didn't want the other moms to see how she was struggling. She thought everyone would judge her and blame her for being a terrible mother.

The constant comparison mothers do at the school and at every event made her become so neurotic about always appearing perfect. The thing was, her life actually was perfect. She had lovely children and a loving husband. Her problem was she couldn't accept the fact that life can have some flaws. It was the constant performance of acting as the perfect wife and mother which made her break down.

After that panic attack, she realized she needed to stop trying so hard all the time. She didn't need to pretend her life was perfect. Once she could let go of this debilitating burden, she realized her life was perfect, just as it was—flaws and all.

Instead of appearing as the best mom, she started spending more time with her kids and stopped doing too much. As a result, her health drastically improved, and she never had another panic attack over something so small. Instead, the small moments in her life became the most important to her, and where she could find some sign of life again.

This book is for moms who are on the verge of a breakdown and for moms who sometimes just need someone to remind them to take care of themselves, too. It's for moms who need someone to relate to—someone to understand them and say, "It's okay. You've got this."

As a mother, you need to tell yourself you deserve to live life to the fullest, just like everyone else. If you are always stressed, always doing chores, and never thinking about anything else, how will you ever be able to find any joy in life?

Reading this book is the first step on your journey to caring more about yourself. Now it's time to put some changes in place to practice the self-care you now know. Start small. Try stopping during the day to take three deep breaths. Then try just a small amount of exercise.

Next, take the kids outside, and be the monster that chases them around the park. If your kids are too old and get embarrassed by you doing that, simply go for a walk. Park the car further away from the school drop-off, so you have to walk for a few minutes. It really can be that easy.

So, this is where I leave you. I know you'll take the information in these pages and put it to good use. And even if you just take on a few tips, you'll change your life for the better.

I wish you love, light, the best of luck in your journey for peace and fulfillment!

REFERENCES

Alisson-Silva, F. Mol Aspects Med. 2016 Oct;51:16-30. https://pubmed.ncbi.nlm.nih.gov/27421909/

Babies born to mothers with sleep apnea have a higher risk of adverse neonatal outcomes: Babies from mothers with sleep apnea more likely to need resuscitation at birth. (2017, June 4). ScienceDaily. https://www.sciencedaily.com/releases/2017/06/170604115749.htm

Barb. (2015, August 7). How Stress affects the body. Health Care Associates & Community CareGivers. https://healthcareassociates.net/how-stress-affects-the-body/

BMJ 2017; 357 doi: https://doi.org/10.1136/bmj.j1957

Davidson, R. J. et al. (2003). Alterations in Brain and Immune Function Produced by Mindfulness Meditation. Psychosomatic Medicine, 65(4), 564–570. https://doi.org/10.1097/01.psy.0000077505.67574.e3

Environmental Working Group Dirty Dozen https://www.ewg.org/foodnews/dirty-dozen.php. Accessed March 2022.

Environmental Working Group Clean Fifteen. https://www.ewg.org/foodnews/clean-fifteen.php. Accessed March 2022

Gardener H. et al. Curr Dev Nutr. 2018 May; 2(5): nzy008. https://pubmed.ncbi.nlm.nih.gov/29555723/

Griffin, R. M. (n.d.). Moms and Sleep Deprivation. WebMD.

https://www.webmd.com/sleep-disorders/features/moms-sleep-deprivation

How to stop overthinking—and start living - Headspace. (n.d.). Stop-Overthinking-Start-Living. https://www.headspace.com/blog/2017/06/01/stop-overthinking-start-living/

Inspiration for the Mind, Body & Soul. (2017, July). http://www.theeternallyhopeful.com/?m=201707

Jennings, K.-A. (2017, April 30). How Magnesium Can Help You Sleep. Healthline. https://www.healthline.com/nutrition/magnesium-and-sleep

Johnson R. K. et al. 10.1161/CIRCULATIONAHA.109.192627. https://pubmed.ncbi.nlm.nih.gov/19704096/

Keng, S.-L et al. (2011). Effects of mindfulness on psychological health: A review of empirical studies. Clinical Psychology Review, 31(6), 1041–1056. https://doi.org/10.1016/j.cpr.2011.04.006

Mann, D. (2021, May 6). What Is RAIN Meditation—and Should You Try It? The Healthy. https://www.thehealthy.com/alternative-medicine/what-is-rain-meditation-and-should-you-try-it/

McClintock, C. H. et al. (2016). Phenotypic Dimensions of Spirituality: Implications for Mental Health in China, India, and the United States. Frontiers in Psychology, 7. https://doi.org/10.3389/fpsyg.2016.01600

McEvoy, C. T. Neurology. April 02, 2019; 92 (14). https://www.ncbi.nlm.nih.gov/pmc/articles/PMC6448450/

McGowan, S. K. et al. (2016). Examining the Relationship Between Worry and Sleep: A Daily Process Approach. Behavior therapy, 47(4), 460–473. https://doi.org/10.1016/j.beth.2015.12.003

McGreevey, S. (2011, January 21). Eight weeks to a better brain. Harvard Gazette; Harvard Gazette. https://news.harvard.edu/gazette/story/2011/01/eight-weeks-to-a-better-brain/

National Institutes of Health. Magnesium fact sheet. Accessed online March 2022. https://ods.od.nih.gov/factsheets/Magnesium-HealthProfessional/

New Book from Center for Creative Leadership Redefines Stress and How to Control It. (2016, November 7). GlobeNewswire News

Room. https://www.globenewswire.com/news-release/2016/11/07/887334/0/en/New-Book-from-Center-for-Creative-Leadership-Redefines-Stress-and-How-to-Control-It.html

Pasha, S. (2020, July 17). Understanding Overthinking And Bidding It A Good-Bye! – The Second Angle. https://thesecondangle.com/understanding-overthinking-and-bidding-it-a-good-bye/

Powell, A. (2018, April 9). Harvard researchers study how mindfulness may change the brain in depressed patients. Harvard Gazette; https://news.harvard.edu/gazette/story/2018/04/harvard-researchers-study-how-mindfulness-may-change-the-brain-in-depressed-patients/

Pregnant mums who snore may affect the reading ability of unborn child. (2017, October 26). NZ Herald. https://www.nzherald.co.nz/nz/pregnant-mums-who-snore-may-affect-reading-ability-of-unborn-child/RLL5JYOCGDGPLGJNLKROU2OEHQ/

Psychology Today. Vitamin C: Stress Buster. Accessed online March 2022. https://www.psychologytoday.com/nz/articles/200304/vitamin-c-stress-buster

Rodrigues, G. S. (2020, October 16). Rumination: When Your Thoughts Don't Have an Off Button. The Psychology Group Fort Lauderdale. https://thepsychologygroup.com/ruminating-thoughts-and-anxiety/

Science Daily. Omega-3 reduces anxiety and inflammation in healthy students, study suggests. Accessed online March 2022. https://www.sciencedaily.com/releases/2011/07/110713121313.htm

Simopoulos, A. P. Biomed Pharmacother 2002 Oct;56(8):365-79. https://pubmed.ncbi.nlm.nih.gov/12442909/

Sizensky, V. (2015, March 27). New Survey: Moms Are Putting Their Health Last. HealthyWomen. https://www.healthywomen.org/content/article/new-survey-moms-are-putting-their-health-last

Sleep apnea - Symptoms and causes. (n.d.). Mayo Clinic. https://www.mayoclinic.org/diseases-conditions/sleep-apnea/symptoms-causes/syc-20377631#:~:text=Sleep%20apnea%20is%20a%20potentially

Spurgeon, D. (2002). People who sleep for seven hours a night live longest. BMJ: British https://www.ncbi.nlm.nih.gov/pmc/ articles/PMC1172056/

The Nutrient Bible. Henry Osiecki. 7th edition. AG Publishing.

ABOUT THE AUTHOR

Zoe Madden is a qualified nutritionist, kinesiologist, engineer, financial planner, writer and editor. This weird combination means she's not only the poster girl for career reinvention, but has a wealth of experience to draw on when it comes to health, wellbeing, and staying sane in this crazy world.

Zoe's passion is honoring mind, body and spirit to bring about balance. She favors clean, green and natural options wherever possible but doesn't advocate rigidly sticking to any particular practice or health regime. She believes what matters most is finding what works for you in this exciting ride that is Motherhood. Her books are intended to be resources to help you do just that.

Visit Zoe at www.zoemadden.com.

Coming Soon

Life is uncertain. What would happen to you and your children if something were to happen to your partner or spouse? Or perhaps you've simply parted or are thinking of parting. Regardless of age or circumstances, nobody wants to be caught out without some form of financial security and knowledge.

Not In His Name: Financial Self-Care for Moms is your guide to financial independence, whether you are married or not. Money isn't everything but it sure helps when it comes to the security, freedom, opportunities and happiness we all deserve.